SITTING KILLS, MOVING HEALS

How Simple Everyday Movement Will
Prevent Pain, Illness, and Early Death —
and Exercise Alone Won't

Joan Vernikos, Ph.D.

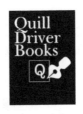

Quill
Driver
Books

Fresno, California

Published by Quill Driver Books
An imprint of Linden Publishing
2006 South Mary Street, Fresno, California 93721
(559) 233-6633 / (800) 345-4447
QuillDriverBooks.com

Quill Driver Books and Colophon are trademarks of
Linden Publishing, Inc.
For permission to use any portion of this book for academic purposes
please contact the Copyright Clearance Center at www.copyright.com.

ISBN 978-1-610350-18-1

Printed in the United States of America
on acid-free paper.

Information contained in this book is not to be construed as medical
guidance. Before beginning any exercise program, consult your physician.

Library of Congress Cataloging-in-Publication Data

Vernikos, Joan.
  Sitting kills, moving heals : how everyday movement will prevent pain,
illness, and early death-- and exercise alone won't / Joan Vernikos.
      p. cm.
  Includes bibliographical references and index.
  ISBN 978-1-61035-018-1 (pbk.)
  1. Exercise. 2. Gravity--Physiological effect. I. Title.
RA781.V47 2011
613.7'1--dc23
                              2011035984

Contents

Acknowledgements

I could not have conceived, written, and gotten this book to this point without the invaluable support, encouragement, and integrity of my husband Geoffrey. My son George's prodding kept me on track, as did endless encouragement from friends Molly Macauley, Dr. Bill Chadduck, and James Pagliasotti. Their suggestions got to the heart of what I was trying to say and were most useful in keeping me focused.

My thanks to my editor Elsa Peterson, who helped me let go of stylistic constraints of years of writing science papers. Her work and encouragement were invaluable. Thank you to Steve Mettee for sensing something worth telling and for the invaluable work, support, and enthusiasm of my publisher and editor Kent Sorsky.

My deepest gratitude and respect go to those remarkable men and women, including the magnificent John Glenn, who volunteered to be test subjects in space or in ground studies. They knew their contribution would help other astronauts remain fit and healthy on their way to Mars. Little did they imagine that their experience would help each one of us remain healthy here on Earth.

Preface

One day in 1997, former astronaut John Glenn walked into my office at the National Aeronautics and Space Administration (NASA) with a pile of notes. At that time, he was chair of the Senate Committee on Aging, and he found himself intrigued by the similarities between his personal experiences in space and my research observations at NASA on the effects of gravity on the human body. Amazingly, Senator Glenn wanted to return to space—but he was eager that his experience should somehow yield practical scientific benefits. I was thrilled to help, and I began to make plans to carefully track his health during and after his flight.

In November 1998, a very fit 77-year-old Glenn made his long-awaited return voyage into space on the shuttle *Discovery*. He was no passenger. He went through the same grueling astronaut training his crewmates did, all while putting in a full schedule in the Senate. And, he carried out his fair share of experiments and assignments during the mission.

Most people are unaware that astronauts who spend much time in space always return home having suffered some degree of physical debilitation. This is because the lack of gravity in space wreaks havoc on the body. Upon Glenn's return, and much to the surprise of most, we found that his body's response to spending nine days in space was indistinguishable from that of his six much-younger crewmates! Had his results been different, his advanced age would naturally have been viewed as the culprit. However, the fact that his condition was the same as the others reinforced our growing belief at NASA that the determining factor in one's ability to withstand and respond to unusual challenges is *not* chronological age—rather, the critical factor is how healthy and active a life one leads

Sadly, our modern sedentary lifestyle—which mimics the lack of gravity experienced by astronauts in space—produces a wide variety of spaceflight-like symptoms, and these problems are becoming apparent at an ever-younger age, and even in children. It wasn't too long ago that the United States government reported more healthy persons than unhealthy. However, recent figures from the Centers for Disease Control and Prevention indicate a stunning 61 percent of the American population is now unhealthy. There has been much debate about our healthcare system, but it is evident that no system can cover the costs of health care when almost every citizen is unhealthy, and at current rates that is where we are heading in the next ten or twenty years.

So let me tell you why I wrote this book. While the country was figuring out who pays for health care, here I was, sitting on a practical, inexpensive, scientifically-proven solution derived from research paid for by the taxpayer! Astronauts, chosen on the basis of being the healthiest and the fittest—of possessing the "right stuff"—are transformed by the lack of gravity in space into the likes of seniors thirty of forty years older. Yet, despite the debilitating effects of spaceflight, astronauts fully recover soon after they return to Earth. Why not use what we have learned about astronauts at NASA to benefit the rest of us?

It became my passion to share, in plain language that anyone could understand, the knowledge we acquired from our research at NASA. If astronauts could regain their good health after shaking off the ill effects of spaceflight, so could people suffering similar health problems due to their sedentary lifestyles. My challenge was to provide clear, practical guidance to show the public the value of making use of our old friend gravity, simply through doing everyday activities that were of a different nature than traditional vigorous exercise in the gym.

Perhaps it's just the facts-loving scientist in me, but I have found people are more likely to persevere in a lifestyle change if they understand *why* what they do matters. I therefore parted ways with agents and publishers who advised me to "just tell people *what* to do"; I needed to explain the "why" of this exciting, life-changing research. This book does just that, in addition to providing an action plan that can give you a lifetime of physical health. Why wait to be sick before you decide to be well?

Here's to your continuing good health!

—Joan Vernikos, Ph.D.

Introduction

Gravity Is Our Friend

When you wake up in the morning, do you feel full of energy? Can you smile at the weather, your children dashing off to school, the dog begging to be taken for a walk? Is there a spring to your step as you look forward to your day's work? If you answer "yes," you are one of the lucky ones. But if you're like most people, you probably have the urge to just plop down in front of the computer or the TV, or maybe even slip into bed for another hour of sleep. The energy just isn't there. You're sluggish. You sometimes wonder if there's something wrong with you? Maybe the doctor could run some tests or give you a pill to take the pain and sluggishness away. All you know is that you're tired of feeling like the weight of the world is resting on your shoulders and aching joints, slowing you down and turning your day into a grind.

Here's something that might surprise you: Did you know that what makes you feel so heavy, tired, and unfit is the same thing that makes the apple fall straight down off the tree? Gravity! You can let it pull you down, as so many of us living sedentary lives quite literally do. Or you can enlist it as a powerful and faithful ally in your efforts to be healthy and feel good. You can use gravity to achieve and sustain good health. It's your choice.

The human body is a wondrous machine. You may think you're sitting still as you read this book. But, in fact, the muscles in your eyes are moving as you read, and nerve impulses are traveling from your eyes to your brain, where additional neural activity enables you to interpret these characters as words, sentences, and ideas. Your heart muscle is beating, circulating blood throughout your body. The capillaries in your lungs are extracting vital oxygen from the air you breathe. Your digestive organs are converting your most recent meal into nutrients that give you energy and renew your cell tissues. Your bones, too, are constantly taking up new calcium from your diet to build and repair themselves. Even your brain's nervous system is in a continual state of renewal. Internally, your body is constantly in motion—if it ever stopped, you'd be dead. Indeed, you might say that the human body is designed to be a perpetual motion machine.

Gravity is the driving force behind all this perpetual motion. Colorless, odorless, tasteless, it's something that those of us who live on Earth have always taken for granted. We cannot see it, though we learn from experience its predictable effects: childhood tumbles, car keys accidentally dropped into a mud puddle, a basketball gracefully curving down toward the hoop. A friend once told me a story about helping her brother with a do-it-yourself carpentry project in which they needed to draw a straight vertical line. She was reaching for a ruler and a level when her more experienced brother said, "Let's let gravity be our friend." He tied a string around his keys, let them drop, and—presto!—there was a straight vertical line. In our physiological makeup, as in carpentry, gravity is our friend. It is gravity that enables our muscles to know they are being used, so that they can rebuild themselves. The same is true for our bones and for our nerve fibers.

Scientists have long known that plants use gravity to grow healthy roots, but nobody knew about gravity's role in keeping the human body healthy until we had the opportunity to observe the one group of people who had ever lived *without* gravity—astronauts. During my thirty years of research, and during and after my time as Director of Life Sciences for NASA, solving this mystery was my passion.

I wrote this book so that I could share with you what has been learned about how the body and brain need to use gravity to remain healthy. Did you know that our brains automatically sense and translate gravity into maps and programs etched into our nervous system, enabling us to move in a coordinated manner? We discovered this by going into space. What this means is that movement is ineffective without gravity, and *gravity is downright harmful unless we move.* Recent research along these lines is helping us develop a profile of how to use gravity to achieve good health. It turns out that the best technique is quite different from the common method of exercising in a gym once a day or several times a week. Rather, a multitude of frequent, low-intensity stimuli, throughout the day, 365 days a year is the optimal approach. In other words, the secret to good health on Earth that space exploration revealed is the need for perpetual motion.

But who says we don't already use gravity? How can we avoid using it, since we are exposed to it every minute of our lives on Earth? This is true; however, humans today use gravity much less than did our ancestors throughout history. Prehistoric people had to move about constantly in order to defend themselves, run away from danger, and hunt and gather food to survive. Human genes evolved over millions of years to meet the requirements of continuous motion, both internally and for the body as a whole. As civilization came into being, humans continued to plough the land, tend animals, cut trees, do heavy work, and move from place to place. They were still in motion.

This changed somewhat during the Industrial Revolution, but the big shift began in the twentieth century. Spurred on by World War II and the Space Age, technological inventions burst into our lives at a breath-taking pace. First it was the automobile, which allowed people to travel farther, faster, and in more comfort than ever before; it also freed tens of thousands from the heavy lifting involved with harnessing, feeding, and cleaning up after horses, which had previously been the principal means of transportation. In the home, automatic washing machines and clothes dryers meant no more struggling with heavy wet laundry, and electric and gas stoves meant no more chopping wood. In the yard and garden, power lawn mowers and leaf blowers replaced manual mowers and rakes. By the mid-1950s, homeowners no longer needed to get out of their cars to open the garage door, and they could sit comfortably at home watching television rather than going out to a movie. By the late 1990s, a trip to the public library or the mall, or even picking up the telephone to communicate, became largely unnecessary, as we became adept at using search engines, online merchants, e-mail, and instant messaging.

Designed to make life easier, these inventions quickly became integral parts of our existence. But what many of us did not realize is that these labor-saving devices have a serious downside: They systematically rob us of all the habitual movements we used to make when we lived without them—the perpetual motion our great-grandparents engaged in, day in and day out, throughout their entire lives. Now, to a far greater degree than our ancestors, we simply sit. And many of us sit pretty much all day long. We sit in our cars and trucks, we sit in our offices, and we go home in the evening and sit in front of the TV or the computer.

The human body is designed to be much more physically active than most of us are today. Yet we have an understandable craving for comfort, and these inventions provide comfort to a degree previously unknown to even the wealthiest humans. As with any craving, our technological addiction leads us on a never-ending spiral of wanting more and more gadgets to do things for us that our ancestors used to do for themselves. As a result, we in the developed world have experienced a huge increase in serious health consequences, such as obesity, diabetes, heart disease, osteoporosis, muscle wasting and arthritis, balance and coordination problems, poor sleep, and a lack of stamina and energy. These disorders, once believed to be consequences of aging, are now appearing much earlier in life, and sometimes even in children. The deep-rooted motivation to survive can now be met without physical work. But our human genes could not keep up with such rapid change in lifestyle, and so we suffer.

The realization of the causal link between modern labor-saving inventions and their detrimental health consequences came from a most unlikely source: space. We have always considered gravity as the foe that drags us down and dreamed of how liberating it would be to float in the weightlessness of space! But when astronauts traveled away from Earth's gravitational pull, those of us at NASA who were monitoring their physical health were in for quite a shock. The absence of gravity for even a few days accelerated the astronauts' physical degeneration. We found changes in their bodies of the kind that we typically associate with aging. Could it be that living without the downward pull of gravity was actually detrimental? We observed that by merely returning to their active lives on Earth, the astronauts could quickly be restored to full fitness. It became obvious that gravity is a greater contributor to good health than anyone had previously thought. We discovered that living without gravity is like being immobilized, since leg muscles, bones, and the brain and spinal programs that regulate our movements are no longer needed and atrophy. Nothing speeds up brain atrophy like immobilization. And here we are, an entire population voluntarily immobilizing itself with its sedentary, comfort-oriented lifestyle. Gravity can't help us when we're sitting!

This book is about how each of us can make friends with gravity. It tells why, when, how often, how much, and exactly how you can make the most effective use of gravity for lifelong health and vigor. You'll learn to prevent the age-related decline that has long been assumed to be inevitable, remain fit and healthy, and even use gravity as therapy for specific health problems.

The key lies not in giving up the comforts and conveniences that modern technology has to offer, but in encouraging the reintroduction of gravity-challenging activities into everyday living. Increasing awareness of gravity in all we do and systematically converting daylong, natural, non-exercise activities into lifelong habits (I call them "G-habits") is the first step to better health. Preventive health care starts at home with a foundation of constant motion to reset and sustain health, strength, confidence, and vigor. If this systems works for the astronauts, it can certainly work for you!

PART ONE:

WHY YOU NEED GRAVITY FOR GOOD HEALTH

1

Gravity 101

The physical deterioration suffered by astronauts in space in a matter of days mirrors what happens to all of us here on Earth as we age. However, living in space profoundly magnifies the changes that normally take a lifetime to appear. On Earth, from age 20 we lose roughly 1 percent of our bone density a year. Yet astronauts in space, on average, lose 1.6 percent of their bone density a month, and some have lost as much as 1 percent in a single week! This is on top of their muscles becoming weaker, their immune systems being suppressed, and their sleep being disturbed. And when they first return from space, they have less stamina, they shuffle when walking, and they have lost their sense of balance. It's tough being an astronaut!

Fortunately, these dramatic changes are reversed after astronauts return home and commence a recovery regimen. So what exactly is their secret to restoring full health? What can we Earth-bound folks learn from the experience of astronauts that can help us keep our own strength and youthful vigor? The answers to these questions form the basis of this book's gravity prescription, and constitute a practical survival kit to wellness right here on Earth.

WHAT HAPPENS TO ASTRONAUTS IN SPACE?

John Glenn's memorable return to space in 1998 on the shuttle *Discovery* once more highlighted the fact that astronauts returning from space show a pattern of symptoms that collectively resemble those seen in older persons. The medical community initially concluded in the early 1970s, when these observations were first made during the Skylab missions, that astronauts grow old faster in space. However, it soon became clear that astronauts fully recover shortly after they return to their normal lives on the ground. Was this a reversal of the aging process? And were astronauts *really* aging more quickly in space?

In order to investigate these questions, NASA scientists had to find a way to simulate the absence of gravity in an experimental condition on Earth. We knew that sitting in water was a possible way to create this simulation—although we aren't quite weightless in water, we do weigh less because the water that our body displaces is pushing back upward against us. But we found we couldn't keep human subjects immersed in water up to their necks for more than a few hours at a time because of "prune skin" and other problems.

After trying a few different conditions, it was determined that simply lying flat on one's back reduced the pull of gravity on the body sufficiently to allow the effects to be studied. This is because, when we lie down, gravity is pulling down only *across* the torso—the depth and width of the body—rather than pulling downward (from head to toe) on the entire body height. In my 30 years of conducting research on this question, I used healthy young men and women volunteers to study the effects of space flight, as closely as could be induced by lying in bed continuously, without getting up to go to the bathroom or for any other reason. What I found is that the same changes that appear in astronauts appeared in the bed-bound volunteers, albeit more slowly. Surely these volunteers couldn't be growing old faster merely by lying in bed!

Like astronauts, the bed-bound research subjects recovered shortly after being up and about. I learned from my research that how quickly they and astronauts recovered largely depended on how many days they had been in bed or in space. For short durations of low-gravity existence, one day of recovery is required for each day spent in bed or in space. However, for gravity-deprived durations beyond 30 days, recovery is slower—more like two and a half days of recovery for every day in space, and even longer for some bodily components, such as bone.

Like others, I had initially believed that advanced age in a subject would further slow down this rate of recovery, but I was proven wrong. In fact, when senior astronauts such as 77-year-old John Glenn and 55-year-old Story Musgrave flew in space, they not only suffered deterioration during spaceflight that was no more severe than what their younger crewmates suffered, but they also recovered just as quickly once back home on

Earth. From this and many other observations and experiments, I arrived at the conclusion that astronauts do not in fact grow older in space. The lack of gravity causes a rapid progression of the kinds of changes in their bodies that we on Earth *associate* with age. But these changes don't come about from merely piling up years of life—these are actually a direct consequence of the sedentary lifestyles we tend to adopt as we get older, lifestyles that don't use the head-to-toe gravity "vector," and instead involve a great deal of sitting.

A PHYSICIST IN SPACE

Stephen Hawking, physicist, mathematician, and best-selling author of *A Brief History of Time* (1988), caught the world's imagination when, at age 65, he floated free of his wheelchair aboard G-Force One, a specially-converted Boeing 727 that flew out of Cape Canaveral. Since his early 20s, the academic celebrity has suffered from motor neuron disease, also known as Lou Gehrig's disease; throughout most of his adult life, he has been almost completely paralyzed. Under the close supervision of a trained team, Hawking levitated eight times for about 20 seconds each—a total of about two-and-a-half minutes in free fall. Communicating through an electronic synthesizer and raised eyebrows, a beaming Hawking said, "The zero gravity bit was wonderful. I could have gone on and on. Space, here I come!"

GRAVITY AND LIFE

Gravity is the force of attraction between two masses. It is a part of nature, a force of the universe. It holds the world together and we are all linked by it. Gravity exerts its stimulating benefits on the human body in many different ways. When you stand upright, you feel the pull of gravity as it pulls you down to Earth. When you are relaxed, you let your body be sucked downward by Earth—this, too, is gravity's work.

Gravity firmly grounds us. It determines how we look, how we function, and what we weigh. It pulls in one direction only: downward. When we stand up, we say we experience one degree of gravity (1G). Therefore, how we orient ourselves toward this invisible, colorless, odorless, silent force determines how we use the gravity vector to stimulate different parts of the body. You can run faster with less effort if you're running downhill because gravity pulls at your body, helping you down. It is gravity that slows you as you try to run uphill away from it.

From the very beginnings of life on Earth and throughout its evolution over the past 3.5 billion years, gravity has been ever-present. Given how pleasant it feels to be free of gravity's downward pull, it is hardly surprising that life forms started out in water, where they are spared gravity's maximum influence. Plants on Earth's surface have limited mobility and use gravity in relatively simple ways. They derive directional cues of up or down, and use gravity to separate and layer their internal components in a way that controls their growth and development.

Whether we are talking about plants, animals, or humans, the gravity vector not only acts on the whole body, but on its component parts as well. Life forms are mostly liquid—you have probably heard it said that the human body is about 75 percent water. How, then, do we keep from sloshing down onto the floor? Our bodies are held in place by physical surfaces, such as cell membranes, that isolate their different constituents. When you stand up, gravity pulls your blood toward your feet, and your heart must pump hard against gravity to send blood back up to your head. Gravity makes particles in a liquid settle, and makes liquids mix or separate, as in salad dressing. Cell structure and function, as well as organ development, were designed so that they would not collapse when pulled down by gravity. The nervous system—which you can think of as the body's intercom system—grew to sense and respond to changes in the environment, like reflexes that make you pull your hand away from a hot stove or go indoors when it is cold. Nerve cells and axons also grew to sense and respond to the gravity vector. Everything was created to support the processes of life and survival.

Living creatures continuously changed to become more complex and sophisticated. As they emerged out of the water, life hedged its bets with gravity. First, as with frogs and their ancestors, they were amphibious, living in both land and water, staying close to the ground and slithering around (or possibly taking the occasional gravity-defying hop into the air). Then, as with dinosaurs, larger life forms evolved stronger bones and musculature that could resist the pull of gravity for hours at a time, enabling them to stand off the ground on four legs and to run faster than amphibians. Eons later, humans began to engage gravity more directly by balancing erect on our "hind" legs and walking about.

Throughout its evolution, life has therefore had to develop, adjust, and adapt to gravity. We might say that it is a constant balancing act between the physiology of the body and the force of gravity, except for the fact that it is a one-sided game: The force of gravity does not change, it is ever-present, so it is the body that must change and adapt. Our body was designed to live in gravity as a perpetual motion machine.

LOSING THE MEMORY OF GRAVITY

Space exploration offers huge potential for better understanding human physiology on Earth, and we have only scratched the surface. Space experiments have shown that balance sensors in the inner ear are tremendously plastic—that is, they adapt readily. In fact, this adaptation to lower gravity stimulation takes place within hours. NASA scientist Muriel Ross showed that, in the absence of gravity, this plasticity takes the form of an

---

A THOUGHT EXPERIMENT

One of my favorite explanations of gravity comes from *Gravity Is a Mystery*, a wonderful children's book written many years ago by Franklyn M. Branley, Astronomer Emeritus and former chairman of the American Museum of Natural History's Hayden Planetarium. The gist of it is that if you dug a hole through the center of the earth and kept digging long enough you would come out in the Indian Ocean (assuming you started somewhere in the continental United States). Now, if you jumped into the hole, you would keep falling faster and faster—you would accelerate—right past the center. Then, because of the momentum you had built up, on the other side of the center, you would fall *up* and away from the center, slowing down until the force of gravity overcame your momentum and you stopped. You would be almost in the Indian Ocean, but not quite. Branley writes: "Now you would fall back toward the center of the earth. You would go faster and faster, right past the center. But you would not quite reach your starting point. Back and forth you would go. Each time, you would go a shorter distance past the center. Back and forth, back and forth. Gravity would make you fall toward the center of the earth. When you moved past the center, gravity would pull you back again. After a long, long time you would stop moving. You would stay at the center of the earth. Gravity pulls you toward the center of the earth."[1]

---

increase in communication sites—synapses of hair cells—lying between the gravity sensor cells and the nerve fibers ending on them.[2] Not surprisingly, the reverse occurs with increased gravity stimulation on a centrifuge, so that the sensors become less sensitive. With continued exposure to the absence of gravity, the stretch and touch sensors (proprioceptors) in the feet are dulled and may completely disappear, though this has not happened yet in astronauts with exposures of up to six months in space.

Hitting the Risk Zone

In our everyday life on Earth, it is easy to give in to gravity. We love the relaxing feeling of lying in bed, curling up on the couch, or floating in a swimming pool. We dislike the effort it takes to rise out of bed, climb out of a car, or carry a bag of groceries into the house. At some point in our 30s or 40s, we look in the mirror and see that our facial muscles and certain contours of our body are not quite as firm and buoyant as we remember them being when we were younger. A friend told me how, at 30, she noticed that the shape of her hips suddenly had a lower curve to it. Although she described this as "not bad, just different," it is the kind of bodily change that throws some of us into a panic. We think of gravity as the enemy that makes everything go south. And, sure enough, it will drag us down if we let it.

So we are advised to exercise, to be active. The way to maintain the resilience of our bodies, we are told, is to use our muscles: Get up out of bed and off the couch, choose a parking space far away from the store's entrance, carry our purchases rather than wheeling them in a cart, etc. And, to a certain extent, this advice is correct.

But we know from space research and bed-rest studies that exercise alone is not the complete answer. Studies have shown that exercise during space or bed-rest was useful, but rarely was it more than 50 percent effective in keeping muscles and bones from wasting. To reset the cardiovascular system after 16 days of deconditioning in bed, you have to pedal at maximal intensity for 15 minutes—and the benefits last only 24 hours. Notice I used the word "maximal." The doctors will not allow the astronauts to exercise maximally while in space because they are concerned about possible arrhythmias; however, exercising sub-maximally, even for longer periods, doesn't seem to do the recuperation trick.

Have you ever performed a stress EKG? This test is structured to build up in increments to maximal effort, and it is pretty unpleasant for most people. Now, imagine keeping up the same pace for 15 minutes. We use it as a test to measure VO^2max, which is aerobic capacity—how many liters of oxygen you can take in relative to the "work" you do. The key here is that only intensity seems to reset the cardiovascular system, or kick it into gear. But it is not easy to pedal as hard as you can for 15 minutes, and it's certainly not the sort of thing one would choose to repeat every 24 hours.

As an aside, after studying this subject for years, I can think of only one example from my experience at NASA that may contradict some of what I've said here. One Russian cosmonaut did come back from a space voyage in good shape. His secret? Well, he quarreled with a fellow cosmonaut and was so angry that he spent a good part of his entire day, every day, on the treadmill so that he would not have to interact with his crewmate. He exercised for as much as eight hours every day! Best thing he ever did. But aren't you glad we live on a planet with gravity so that we can stay in shape without having to do *that* much work? Movement is valuable, but the presence of gravity is crucial for it to be effective.

It has often been said that every one of us will either grow old or die young—there is no third choice. However, if we are fortunate enough to avoid an early death and grow old chronologically, will we inevitably suffer the deterioration of our bones, muscles, and nervous system that are traditionally associated with aging? If you are young and healthy as you read this, stop for a moment and ask yourself these questions: How old do you want to be before you lose the ability to ski or ride a bicycle? How old do you want to be before you lose bone density to the point where a fall on the sidewalk could result in a hip fracture? How old do you want to be before you have to wear special undergarments because you no longer have good bladder control? If you are like most people, you would like to postpone reaching this point—what I call the "risk zone"—as long as you can.

Most of us have seen older people whose posture is stooped, who walk unsteadily, too weak to sit down or stand up without help. When one reaches this stage of physical decline, it becomes difficult or impossible to live independently, and it is the loss of independence that people approaching their retirement years hate to contemplate. In a survey of more than 8,000 older adults, Australian researchers Susan Quine and Stephen Morrell learned that "Apart from the fear of losing one's physical health, the participants' main fear...was of losing their independence, with a specific fear of nursing home admission."[3]

Health, indeed life itself, is at risk when we lose our independence. In one study, researchers in the Finnish Centre for Interdisciplinary Gerontology followed more than 1,000 older adults for a period of eight years. They divided these adults into three categories: those who were fully mobile and active, those who had some impairment but were active nevertheless, and those who were impaired and sedentary. At the end of eight years, they found that "In men and women, the relative risk of death was two times greater in Impaired-Active and three times greater in Impaired-Sedentary groups than was the risk of death in Mobile-Active groups."[4]

In other words, those who had normal mobility were more likely to be alive eight years later than those who had impaired mobility, and the mobile-impaired adults who exercised were more likely to be alive than the mobile-impaired adults who led sedentary lives.

My friend Tom Rogers said, "I want to be healthy and independent till I drop dead," and I agree with him! If reaching the risk zone means losing my health and independence, I want to drop dead before I reach that stage. The vote is universal when I ask about this at my talks: We all want to postpone reaching the risk zone as long as possible.

If, from the age of 20, you lose 1 percent bone density a year under normal ambulation circumstances, you will likely hit the risk zone in your 80s. The ultimate gravity deprivation that one experiences in space amplifies this rate of change to 1–2 percent per *month*. Muscle is similar—1 percent per year on Earth versus 1 percent per month in space. Even on Earth, a reduction to less than average activity—as in a lifestyle that involves an excessive amount of sitting—would accelerate your reaching the risk zone, so that if you are very sedentary you may reach the risk zone in your 40s or 50s. If we are not careful, we can start to suffer changes in balance as early as the 20s, as can happen when young women wear high heels and go down a flight of stairs looking at their feet and holding onto the railing. In contrast, the risk zone can be delayed—or even reversed, as it was in Maria Fiatarone's 1994 study with men and women as old as 90 at the Hebrew Rehabilitation Center in Boston. Working with colleagues from Tufts University, they showed that 12 weeks' training with weights increased muscle strength and endurance, and even restored bone density.[5]

This is what I am talking about when I say that the use of gravity determines how fast we age, not in years, but at what age we hit the risk zone.

THE MECHANICS OF GRAVITY

If you're interested in a technical explanation of how gravity works, read on! Particles and objects have mass. These objects could be stars in the universe, the apple that Sir Isaac Newton famously observed falling from a tree, or our very own bodies. Stars and planets maintain their relative positions in the universe by virtue of their gravitational field and their mass. Gravity depends not only on mass and distance, but also density and other factors, so calculating the gravity force of a given body is a fairly complex operation. But it's easy to remember this: Gravity is quantified in Gs, and we stipulate that Earth has a gravity of 1G. Our moon has a smaller mass and a gravity force that is only 0.16G. Mars, with a diameter about half that of Earth and a position in the solar system considerably farther from the sun than Earth's, has a gravity force of 0.32 G, roughly one third that of Earth.

Earth attracts our body mass and pulls us towards its center. It is this pull of gravity that gives weight to our bodies. It is also what gives us a strong sense of direction. Any time we move and reposition ourselves, we expose a different part of our body to gravity's force.

Gravity is also a force of acceleration (the increase in velocity of our movement). Bob Phillips, a backup astronaut, describes it to his students this way: If you jumped from an airplane without a parachute, you would travel 9.8 meters the first second, twice as far the next second, and so on until air resistance slows your rate of acceleration and, gradually, stops it, at which point you would continue falling at a constant speed. Eventually, your free fall would be stopped by the ground, where you would crash from the impact of your accumulated G-load—unless your fall was slowed down by a parachute. Here's another example: If you jumped as high as you could off the ground, you might land with an impact as great as 6G, or six times your body weight, putting significant strain on your legs and ankles, which would have to absorb the impact.

When Neil Armstrong and Buzz Aldrin landed on the moon in 1969, images sent to Earth showed them hopping around in what looked like slow motion. The greatly decreased gravity on the moon meant their acceleration was much, much slower. It also meant that they could leap high into the air with very little effort. Imagine what kinds of records athletes might someday set in a Lunar Olympics!

Chapter 1 Notes

1. Branley, F. M. *Gravity Is a Mystery*. New York: Thomas Y. Crowell, 1986.

2. Ross, M. D. "Gravity Sensor Plasticity in the Space Environment". NASA-Ames Research Center. http://astrobiology.arc.nasa.gov/workshops/1996/astrobiology/speakers/ross/ross_abstract.html ; see also Ross, M.D., "A spaceflight study of synaptic plasticity in adult rat vestibular maculas". *Acta Oto-Laryngologica*, Supplementum 516:1–14, 1994.

3. Quine, S., Morrell, S. "Fear of loss of independence and nursing home admission in older Australians." *Health & Social Care in the Community*. Blackwell Publishing, 15(3): 212–220(9), May 2007.

4. Hirvensalo, M., Rantanen, T., Heikkinen, E. "Mobility difficulties and physical activity as predictors of mortality and loss of independence in the community-living older population." *J Amer Geriatric Soc* 48(5):393–498, 2000.

5. Fiatarone, M., O'Neill, E. F., Ryan, D., Clements, K. M., Solares, G. R., Nelson, M. R., Roberts, S. B., Kehayas, K. K., Lipsitz, L. A., Evans, W. J. "Exercise training and nutritional supplementation for physical frailty in very elderly people." *NEJ Med*, 330:1769–1775, 1994.

2

Gravity Deprivation Syndrome

In my job at NASA, my first concern was to provide knowledge and tools to keep astronauts healthy while they lived and worked in space. If we could succeed at that, maybe one day the average person of the future would be able to travel on a spacecraft, just as they do today on ships and airplanes. Rather than going on an adventure holiday to the Amazon or Antarctica, we might take a trip to the moon!

The Space Race made it possible for the first time to understand how the force of gravity we live with here on Earth determines how we look, feel, and function. In a spacecraft, we provide an Earth-like environment for astronauts to live in, but with insignificant gravity. It's the perfect place to conduct gravity deprivation research.

However, determining how astronauts could maintain their health in space was no easy task. Before the Space Age, scientists predicted dire consequences would result from thrusting a human being into weightless flight. Often, these predictions contradicted each other. Various specialists said that the heart would race or that it would stop, that a person would be unable to sleep or would sleep constantly, that an astronaut would become euphoric or profoundly depressed. It was said that the bones would soften, that eating would be impossible, and that the ability to think would be impaired. So acute was the concern for the unknown medical effects of weightlessness that numerous animals were flown, first in ballistic suborbital "zero-G" trajectories, and then finally in complete Earth orbits before either Yuri Gagarin or Alan Shepard first flew their Vostok and Mercury spacecrafts. Happily, most of the predicted dangers did not occur. Weightlessness in general appeared to be surprisingly tolerable. Though some significant changes in the human body were noted even in the earliest flights, as long as astronauts remained in space, they were not affected by their weaker muscles and bones or their inability to keep their balance, because they did not need to use them until they returned to earth. How serious these changes are in the long run continues to be the subject of intense investigation by space medicine specialists around the world. Nevertheless, there was much we had not thought about, and much more research had to be done. Little did I imagine this research would lead me right back home to Earth—to the link between gravity and a good, long, healthy, active life.

THE CONSEQUENCES

No sooner did the first astronauts return from spaceflight than they started complaining of faintness. Wally Schirra, returning from his nine-hour Mercury 8 mission in 1962, called it "feeling woozy." Some even passed out when they first stood up. Here were young, extremely physically fit military men, and their legs suddenly looked thin and spindly. Standing on the deck of the recovery ship (as you may remember, the astronauts used to splash down in the ocean and wait to be fished out), astronaut Pete Conrad was horrified when his friends looked at him and called him "Chicken Legs!"

A decade later, the three Skylab missions in the early 1970s gave us a better chance to study the health of astronauts, because those missions lasted from 28 to 84 days and were specifically designed for biomedical research. With these longer periods, and over the subsequent years on the shuttle and the International Space Station, we were able to study bones, muscles, sleep, and metabolism.[1] What emerged was an astonishing mix of symptoms that characterized living in space; these are summarized in Table 1 in order of typical detectable appearance.

FORGETTING HOW TO LIVE IN GRAVITY

The changes listed in Table 1 vary with the duration of the stay in space; for a short stay, they are relatively minor, but the longer the person stays in space, the more pronounced they become. When astronauts return home to Earth's gravity, we find that even more problems show up; these are listed in Table 2: Symptoms after Returning from Space. Astronauts' bodies, after returning from even a few days in space, are compromised,

TABLE 1: HOW THE BODY CHANGES IN SPACE

- "Moon face"; swollen face, no wrinkles, expressionless
- Space sickness or "stomach awareness"
- Growing taller by 1–1.5 inches as spine lengthens
- Things take longer to do as movement and reaction time are slowed
- Achilles reflex weaker
- Blood volume reduced
- Less thirsty
- Body weight and mass decrease
- Dehydration relative to Earth
- Increased calcium excretion
- Increased risk of kidney stones
- Heart shrinks; cardiac output decreased
- Heart muscle wall becomes thinner
- Red blood cells reduced; erythropoietin reduced
- Stamina/aerobic capacity decreased
- Exercise almost ineffective
- Lowered growth hormone response to exercise
- Body temperature regulation disturbed
- Muscle atrophy; loss of muscle mass
- Muscle strength reduced; size of fibers decreased
- Fat moves in to replace lost muscle
- Muscle sensitivity to insulin reduced
- Muscles less able to take up sugar
- Senses of taste and hearing dulled
- Biological rhythms disturbed

- Sleep disturbed; sleep not restorative
- Calcium lost from bone
- Bone mass and density decreased
- Delayed bone fracture healing
- Gut absorption decreased; affects calcium, drugs
- Gut motility affected; transit time slower
- Increased risk of bladder infection
- Immune system depressed
- Delayed wound healing
- Flare ups of eye and gum infections
- Flare ups of dormant viral infections, e.g., herpes
- Antibiotic effectiveness reduced
- Testosterone reduced

having become maladapted for living on Earth. Unlike the physical changes that occur in space, whose onset is gradual and fairly sequential, the earth-return problems appear all at once.

Among the most serious are problems of posture and locomotion. Sixty-six percent of returning astronauts have difficulty walking in a straight line, and 69 percent report feeling clumsy. About 69 percent also have persistent sensation aftereffects, such as running into a wall when they take a turn or feeling that they are sliding off the foot of the bed when they try to sleep. About 30 percent suffer from vertigo while standing or walking; they feel nauseated and may even vomit. Their head is unstable because their neck muscles have atrophied. Since they did not need to walk in their spacecraft, their sense of balance is out of practice and they walk using short, wide steps, like a toddler. They also have a tendency to drag their toes before putting their foot down, which makes them prone to tripping.

For this reason, and to avoid injuries during their recovery from the flight, astronauts' balance and coordination are tested thoroughly upon their return. One of these tests includes using a small "sway platform" that

TABLE 2: SYMPTOMS AFTER RETURNING FROM SPACE

- Everything feels *very* heavy
- Nausea/possible vomiting
- Spine compressed; back pain
- Standing can lead to fainting
- Blood pressure regulation disturbed
- Decreased cardiac output and stroke volume of the heart
- Reduced stamina
- Reduced strength
- Muscles no longer support spine
- Risk of muscle injury
- Balance disturbed; unsteadiness
- Wide stance; shorter steps
- No sensation of falling
- Walking and coordination problems
- Arms are not projected outward to protect from fall
- Turning corners is challenging
- Tender soles; at first drag feet; tripping is possible
- Loss in peripheral vision when walking
- Disturbed sleep; feel as if slipping off bed
- Feel jet-lagged, tired
- High risk of kidney stones

can gently move forward and backward. I well remember watching astronaut Rick Searfoss in December 1993 standing on this sway platform being tested for balance after 14 days in space. I was horrified as, with eyes shut, he fell forward without even putting his arms out because he did not realize he was falling. We all ran to catch him. Since then, astronauts wear a support harness to protect them from falling during this test.

In space, without gravity, their sense of balance does not tell astronauts where their bodies are, so they must rely on their eyes. Their balance system, which gets no input, is stepped down, while their eyes, given more practice, are stepped up, letting the astronauts know where they are with respect to their surroundings. When they return to earth, their inner ear has forgotten how to react appropriately to gravity, so they have no sensation of falling. Though astronauts seem to recover within a few weeks, symptoms may recur unpredictably and intermittently, increasing the risk of falls during running or while going up or down stairs, and of having accidents while driving a car. Some of the astronauts have gone jogging a couple of days after they returned, only to end up with a muscle injury, much like what might happen to an athlete who has not trained for a while. When we are out of shape, we know that we must work slowly and gradually to avoid injuries and recapture and build our level of fitness. Much to their surprise, astronauts discover that, despite decades of experiences as competent Earthlings, their bodies have already forgotten how to live in gravity!

For space flights of 14 days, the time needed to recover is approximately one day of recovery for every day in space. It takes longer—about two and a half times longer—with stays greater than three months in space. As astronauts go into space for periods of several months, we are finding that some body systems, like bone and muscle, take even longer than two and a half times the length of the time spent in space. Astronaut Clay Anderson admitted in an interview with *Florida Today* that even after intense exercise for two and a half hours a day for 147 of his 152 days on the International Space Station, he "needed several weeks back on Earth to feel normal" again. He "learned that just exercising his body's big muscle groups left the smaller ones, such as those along his spine, weakened from a lack of use."[2]

How Can We Be Deprived of Gravity on Earth?

By assembling this picture of the consequences of gravity deprivation in astronauts, I in time realized that I had come across this mix of symptoms, or "syndrome," before. They are common features we identify with someone old and frail, someone who is bedridden because of an injury or suffering from a wasting disease such as AIDS/HIV or a long-term infection.

In 1997, a list of the "Physiological Changes in Sedentary Adults" was published in *American Fitness* magazine. The following is an approximate comparison of this list with the changes we observe in astronauts in space:

TABLE 3: SEDENTARY ADULTS VERSUS ASTRONAUTS	
Astronauts in Space	**Changes on Earth with Age**
Aerobic capacity decreases by 25% in 7–14 days	Aerobic capacity decreases 10% per decade
Plasma volume decreases by 10–20% in 7–90 days	Plasma volume decreases by 0.5–1% per decade
Bone density decreases by up to 5% per month[3]	Bone density decreases by 1% per year
Muscle mass decreases by 1% per month	Muscle mass decreases by 1% per year
Muscle strength proportionately reduced	Muscle strength proportionately reduced
Flabby muscles	Flabby muscles
Fetal/curved stance	Stooped posture
Reduced force, explosive power	Reduced force, explosive power
Abnormal reflex patterns	Abnormal reflex patterns
Increased fatigability	Increased fatigability
Decreased cardiac output	Decreased cardiac output
Decreased heart stroke volume	Decreased heart stroke volume
Slower movement and reaction time	Slower movement and reaction time
Increased body fat replaces muscle	Increased body fat replaces muscle
Reduced sensitivity to insulin	Reduced sensitivity to insulin
Decreased testosterone	Decreased testosterone
Decreased growth hormone	Decreased growth hormone
Aching joints	Aching joints
Loss of collagen	Loss of collagen

Tender soles on return from space	Tender soles on getting out of bed
Sluggish gut, slower gut transit time and absorption, possible urinary incontinence in women post-flight	Sluggish gut, slower gut transit time and absorption, urinary incontinence

There are, of course, some differences between what we find in sedentary adults versus what astronauts experience. For example, after approximately 270 days in space, muscle remains stable at about two thirds of its initial mass. However, performance continues to decrease. It is not too broad a generalization to say that space accelerates the changes we normally associate with aging.

But, as many astronauts have gone on to live long lives on Earth decades after going into space, and we have continued to monitor their health, we have observed that they do not actually grow old any faster just because they have been in space. They do not die any younger than the rest of us, nor do they suffer from common diseases of aging at younger ages than the general population. Above all, astronauts recover.

GRAVIPAUSE

We all know about menopause—the cessation of a woman's reproductive cycles. It starts when the ovaries act up before their hormones dwindle, and it brings on a variety of changes, such as weight gain, hot flashes and night sweats, emotional irritability, increased bone loss, loss of skin elasticity, and vaginal dryness. Menopause has been the butt of many jokes and is even the subject of a musical comedy.

However, there's another "pause" to be aware of, and this one affects men, too: gravipause. Its signs may appear even in our early 20s, just after our physical development peaks. Gravipause contributes to diabetes, high blood pressure, heart problems, stroke, balance and coordination problems, muscle wasting, and severe bone loss or fracture. These conditions sometimes show up even in teenagers. But in contrast to menopause, it is possible to defer gravipause and ward off its consequences.

Gravipause brings on the negative health changes we see in astronauts deprived of gravity. These problems show up whether you are an astronaut in space, spend a considerable amount of time in bed or just sitting, or you have had a spinal cord injury or some other paralyzing condition such as polio, cerebral palsy, or Lou Gehrig's disease. They also show up if you are an older person with limited mobility, or at any age if you choose to lead a sedentary life. In all cases, whether you become less exposed to gravity or cannot sense or respond to gravity, the same mix of changes develop. The end result is always frailty.

The magnitude of these changes depends on *its onset, how little gravity you use, and how long you remain sedentary.*

LIVING AND WORKING IN SPACE

Going into space requires being launched away from Earth's atmosphere and its gravity. Once the spacecraft orbits around Earth, the effect of gravity is miniscule. Astronauts are therefore essentially weightless, since it is gravity that imparts weight to all things on Earth.

You probably realize that there is no up or down in space. But have you thought about what that means for astronauts, and for the engineers who design spacecraft? Though the interior of a spacecraft is designed with a floor and a ceiling, this is meaningless to astronauts when they are in space. Without gravity, their inner ear senses no direction. However, they quickly learn to rely on visual cues to know where they are and what they are doing.

In order to work in front of a computer console, astronauts need to secure their feet to the floor. If they use a tool or a pen, it will remain suspended wherever they left it until they want to use it again. They can put their trousers on both legs at a time. When they try to exercise on a treadmill, they need to tether themselves with bungee cords or else they could find themselves on the ceiling.

To sleep while aboard the space shuttle, astronauts attached a sleeping bag somewhere in the vehicle. On the International Space Station, small individual compartments were designed for them to slide into, affording more quiet and privacy. Russian cosmonaut and cardiologist Oleg Atkov, who spent six months in space, complained that the worst part of his flight experience was not feeling the weight of his head on his pillow, a feeling we all take for granted when we lay our head down to sleep. He complained that although he slept enough hours, he would not wake up feeling refreshed.

The Slippery Slope Can Start in Your Twenties

We start using gravity less whenever development peaks—on average at around age 20. Think of how active and energetic you were as a child: running, jumping, skipping rope, swinging on a swing, hanging upside down. Then, as an active teenager, you may have spent many hours playing football, baseball, tennis, swimming, followed by partying into the wee hours! But, for the typical adult in a so-called developed country, what follows high school graduation is work or college. With that comes hours of sitting. The average office worker spends six hours a day sitting. There's also sitting while studying or attending classes, and perhaps additional hours each day sitting in front of the television or computer at home. Often laden with new worries and responsibilities, such as taking care of their own needs, or the needs of others—remembering when to do what, attending to food, lodging, laundry—the level of activity for the young adult takes a nosedive. Add to that cheap, readily available food that is not home-cooked—food unavoidably high in sugars and fats—and the slippery slope toward gravipause becomes steeper every day.

In the last century, symptoms of Gravity Deprivation Syndrome (GDS) first became obvious after age 50. As a child, I remember thinking people in their 30s and 40s were old. AARP, when first formed in 1958, defined a senior at age 55. Using more sensitive techniques, we can now detect subtle GDS changes as early as in the 20s.

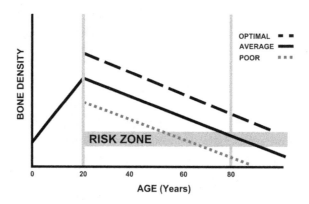

Fig. 1. Hypothetical bone density changes as a function of age
(Adapted and used with permission from Alexandre Kalachi, WHO)

If, for instance, we use bone density loss as a measure of GDS, the chart above, showing average bone loss at the rate of 10 percent per decade, indicates that you would reach the risk zone somewhere around age 80. Apart from genetics, which contribute probably only 20 percent to the formula, those who do not reach the risk zone until 100 are doing something right. What is important in this chart is the *rate* of development of GDS changes, because that determines when you will hit the risk zone—the level that could threaten your quality of life and your independence.

Both in space and in bed rest, the heart muscle atrophies as well. Not unlike the rate of loss of skeletal muscle in space or bed, studies have shown that the heart muscle of intensive care patients can lose 1 percent of heart muscle per week.[4] The calculated loss of cardiovascular function in three weeks of lying in bed in young men, as measured by their aerobic capacity (VO^2max), is equivalent to that seen in those of over 30 to 40 years of aging.[5]

But here's some good news: You can slow down this rate. It's in your hands…and in your legs and in your head! The sooner you start, the better. *It is never too late.* If that doesn't get you out of your chair, I don't know what will!

A BETTER WORLD THROUGH GRAVITY

In the 1950s, modern "conveniences"—the very inventions that, we now know, deprived us of gravity-using activities—were often advertised with phrases like "A Better World through Automation" and "A Better World through Engineering." As you can probably tell if you have read this far, I have a vision of a better world through *gravity*.

How urgent is the need to improve the situation? As just one example, let's look at the public health problem of obesity and related disorders like diabetes. About two thirds of the U.S. population is overweight or obese, with nearly half of that number—almost one third of the population—being obese. (The distinction between the two is based on BMI [body mass index]; an overweight person has a BMI of 25 to 29.99 and an obese person has a BMI of 30 or greater.)

Today, some 26 million Americans—more than 8.3 percent of the total population—are diabetic. At least 79 million Americans—35 percent of adults aged 20 and older—have high blood sugar in the pre-diabetic category.[6] Worse still is the substantial number of cases of diabetes turning up in persons under 20 and in children, not only in the United States, but in other western countries as well. The rate of increase in new cases is getting steeper.[7] Diabetes is not a stand-alone disease. Closely linked to obesity, it doubles the risk of heart disease and stroke. Blindness, kidney failure, and poor circulation requiring amputations are common sequels. Genetic predisposition notwithstanding, both obesity and diabetes are linked to poor eating and sedentary habits. The past 20 years have seen dramatic increases in obesity. In 2010, one third of U.S. adults were obese. What's worse is that 17 percent of children and adolescents aged 2 to 19 years old (12.5 million) are obese. Overall, 64 percent of the American population is either obese or overweight.[8] For many, physical inactivity sadly leads to social inactivity or isolation. But both physical and social inactivity can be countered by adopting an active lifestyle.

How Astronauts Eat

When astronauts eat a meal, they strap their tray to their thigh. Foods are dehydrated to conserve space and prevent spoilage, and they are packed in individual-serving-sized, vacuumed plastic pouches. The astronauts inject water to reconstitute the foods and either suck the food out (if sufficiently liquid) or chew off precut bite-sized portions. I have tried the creamed spinach, which is a favorite, as is the steak and stew. The meal tray also has wells with overlapping plastic covers, because the last thing you want is floating food or crumbs in the spacecraft—something that actually happened in 1965 when a Gemini astronaut, John Young, sneaked a corned beef sandwich on board and offered it to the command pilot, Gus Grissom. What you now take for granted as dehydrated food prepared for your camping trip went through many stages of development over the 45 years of the Space Age.

Because weightlessness makes it impossible to rinse one's mouth out—the water would fly around the room—edible toothpaste had to be developed. For similar reasons, space engineers needed to invent a dry shampoo that would cleanse the scalp without having to be rinsed or brushed out. When astronauts use the toilet, a restraint holds their legs down to prevent them from floating away—ah, the magic of Velcro!

Another less discussed consequence of a sedentary lifestyle is the pelvic muscle weakening that results in urinary incontinence (UI). According to the U.S. Department of Health and Human Services, one in four women age 30–59 have experienced at least one episode of urinary incontinence, a problem we usually associate with old age.[9] Muscle tightening isometric exercises, called Kegels, and vertical acceleration activities such as jumping and dancing can help relieve or eliminate the problem.

Yet an active lifestyle is precisely what is discouraged by the many "modern conveniences" we have come to rely on. Imagine for a moment that this technological trend continues for a few more decades, removing us further from the influence of gravity. What will life be like? I imagine myself waking up one morning and never having to leave my electronic bed. Thanks to information technology advances, I work from home, and it is easy to home-school the children. As I lie comfortably in bed, the mechanisms to draw the curtains and turn on the news on the TV respond to my voice commands. A cheerful robot (probably named Joan in our house) brings in the breakfast tray with piping hot coffee, fruit, cereal, and vitamins. Next come a selection of pads to clean the hands and face, and to lightly exfoliate to keep skin youthful, followed by an electric toothbrush and edible toothpaste. Robot Joan gives good facials and massages as well.

Today's tutoring is on DVD for the children. The horizontal computer terminal swings over the bed. I check on the children via nanny-cam and then it's time to get to work. A meeting will be starting soon: I have to fix my hair, put on a bit of make-up, make a few calls, send messages, and get prepared before I switch on the two-way video. When the meeting is over, I order groceries to be delivered later. Robot Joan brings lunch. Back on the computer, I check the children's schoolwork and plan my work for the afternoon. The children move on to an hour of Game Boy playtime, then virtual soccer. Then it's exercise time for me—Robot Joan helps me slide the horizontal bicycle over the bed for a ride through virtual woods. After dinner, I enjoy a game of bridge with friends by video-link or maybe some virtual tennis or an interactive movie. And, when I absolutely need to get out of bed, I press a button and my electronic bed will lift me gently onto my feet so that I do not faint, just like today's lift chair does. An unlikely scenario? For many, such a lifestyle would be very tempting.

We have the option to reverse this tide. How? By becoming aware of the negative health impacts of these technological "blessings" and by taking action. We cannot turn back the clock back to the nontechnological past, nor should we want to. But good things never come without consequences.

When I was growing up, we would spend summers on Sifnos, a small Greek island in the Aegean. Before electric power arrived, my sister and I would fight every morning over who was to pump rain water collected in the cistern below the house to the metal storage tank on the roof, where the sun provided free heating. We got stronger doing what was fun. Fast-forward to the 1990s: KickStart, a San Francisco organization dedicated to sustainable economic growth in developing countries, developed a line of leg-powered water pumps to provide irrigation for farms of up to two acres. With one of these pumps, not only is a family protected from the risk of inadequate rainfall, they also get the bodybuilding benefits of working the pump. What a wonderful eco-friendly example of the "better world through gravity" concept!

Another example is something my cousin discovered accidentally when she was trying to appease her bored, frail, 94-year-old mother by thinking up something to keep her busy. She handed her mother a bag of almonds and a nutcracker, not really expecting her to be able to manage the task. The housebound lady took on the challenge. She derived immense satisfaction from filling a bag with fresh-shelled almonds, which she then gave to visiting friends. The negative part of this activity was that my cousin could hardly keep up providing her with almonds. The positive benefits were that as word got around, the mother received more visitors—and, thanks to the increased use of muscles in her arms, she could now raise herself from her chair without help.

Let me assure you that I am not here to tell you to give up your indoor plumbing, your easy chair, or your favorite kitchen gadget. However, my vision of a better world does involve a change in the direction our society is headed. My vision involves daily habits that allow us to use gravity for our benefit, and it changes the way our environment is built to encourage these positive habits. Think of the last time you used a multilevel parking garage: Was there a well-lit stairway available, or were people expected to use an elevator to get to and from their cars? In offices, are workers expected to stay seated for hours at a time without leaving their desks? At the hardware store, can you find a good quality leaf rake or snow shovel, or does the store emphasize a selection of power leaf and snow blowers? If you play golf, do you carry your own clubs, or does your course encourage you to use a cart? Look around the supermarket and compare the aisles devoted to frozen dinners and other prepared foods versus the displays of fresh produce and ingredients for cooking from scratch. Sometimes it is not just convenience that gets in the way of an active lifestyle, it's the law—many residential communities have regulations forbidding the use of outdoor clotheslines, ignoring the fact that hanging laundry on a clothesline saves energy while at the same time provides beneficial gravity-based exercise for the body.

My vision of a better world through gravity also involves today's children, who are tomorrow's adults. In today's world, where the safety of children is of prime concern, the freedom to walk to school alone, or to play outdoors or in playgrounds on their own, is something many children never experience. Many children ride to school because of mandatory busing. It is generally the low-income minority children who are bused to the schools in the suburban neighborhoods, not the other way around. When the low-income children get home, they are not allowed outdoors because the streets are unsafe. Sitting indoors watching TV or playing Game Boy begins to look like a pretty good idea when the alternative is getting roughed up or being recruited by older kids in gangs. Today, when many of us need some housekeeping or gardening done, we don't think of involving our children. We think, "Who can I hire to do it?" Our next generation of adults is growing up headed for the risk zone at an early age. The impact of this trend is too serious to be ignored. It is our responsibility to intervene.

In the remaining chapters of this book, you'll find some positive steps you can take to make better use of gravity in your own life, as well as learn ways gravity can be helpful as therapy for those with specific health problems. It is time to make a change.

Getting Inspiration from Children

Like an adult stepping out of a hot tub, babies emerging from the buoyancy of their mother's womb show all the signs of GDS. In their case, it is not a question of relearning how to use gravity. They have never experienced it, so they have to learn from scratch how to use gravity in order to live in it. They have to develop the sensors to sense it and the nerve networks to respond to it. Through a process of action and feedback, appropriate movements they might make instinctively tell their brain during that critical early period of life to lay down nerve networks. Through trial and error, these networks grow and become programmed until they become coordinated and respond appropriately throughout their adult life.

When first born, babies cannot hold their heads up. They need three to four weeks of living in gravity to build up the muscles in the back of the neck to support the head. Their arms gradually become stronger so that by about four or five months they can push themselves up; at six months, they are ready to experience gravity's pull on their upper bodies as they become able to sit upright. Meanwhile, their legs have been gaining in strength. At around seven months, babies begin to crawl, which involves using their legs to push their bodies forward at right angles to the pull of gravity. Soon the leg muscles are strong enough to hold the body upright in a standing position, although the baby still needs to hold onto people or furniture for balance. Some time around 10 to 14 months, babies begin to walk, initially holding their feet wide apart for balance—just like John Glenn returning from his second flight on the shuttle—then gradually with their feet closer together. Babies taking their first steps do a lot of tripping and falling, but they soon learn to bend their knees against gravity, picking each foot up high enough to take longer steps and avoid tripping. Then there is no stopping them as they run, hop, jump, tumble, cartwheel, handstand, hang upside down, seemingly with endless energy!

We adults have much to learn about how to use the gravity vector by watching children. Nobody teaches a child how to use it. They do it instinctively. They stretch when they wake up, much like cats and dogs. They learn to grasp hold of the weight of a cup and guide it to their mouth. And, later on, the games they choose to play are specifically suited to make maximum use of the gravity vector in stimulating growth and development: running, climbing, hopping, skipping, jumping, turning somersaults and cartwheels, swinging on a swing, skipping rope, playing hopscotch, spinning, climbing on bars, hanging with the head down, crawling in and out of any small space, sliding down a slide, wrestling, throwing or hitting or kicking a ball. Later, learning to swim, surf, row, ride a bicycle, ski, skate, ride roller-coasters make up more of their repertory.

What's more, children derive great excitement and pleasure from these gravity-stimulating activities. Their peals of laughter and song tell us that play is fun. The variety of activities they choose reflects the many ways the gravity vector works on the body. Sport may continue until development peaks, or maybe development peaks when activity dwindles. Whatever the reason, why not continue to play and have fun throughout adulthood? *Why not at least carry on with activities you can still master and enjoy?*

Shakespeare astutely observed that old age is like a second childhood, only "sans teeth, sans eyes, sans taste, sans everything." Both conditions share similarities: babies because they have never experienced gravity, the old because they have quit using it. The outcome is the same whether you are in space, living in the almost complete absence of gravity, or lying continuously in bed, where the effectiveness of gravity is reduced, or if you go through life neglecting to use gravity. By the time we are considered old, we have a full-fledged case of GDS, just like astronauts.[10] It doesn't have to be that way. Why not take action to prevent this sorry outcome?

Chapter 2 Notes

1. Vernikos, J. "Human Physiology in Space," *BioEssays*, 18:1029–1037, 1996.

2. *Florida Today* (2/6/08, Peterson).

3. Keyak, J. H., Koyama, A. K., LeBlanc, A., Lu Y., Lang, T. F. "Reduction in proximal femoral strength due to long-durationspaceflight." *Bone* 2009, 44(3):449–453.

4. Perhonen, M. A., Franco, F., Lane, L. D., Buckey, J. C., Blomquist, C. G., Zerwe, K. H. J. E., Peshok, R. M., Weatherall, P. T., Levine, B. D. "Cardiac atrophy after bed-rest and space flight." *J Appl Physiol* 91:645–653, 2001.

5. McGavock, J. M., Hastings, J. L., Snell, P. G., McGuire, D. K., Pacini, E. L., Levine, B. D., Mitchell, J. H. "A forty-year follow-up of the Dallas bed rest and training study: the effect of age on the cardiovascular response to exercise in men." *J Gerontol A Biol Sci Med Sci* 64A(2): 293–299, 2009.

6. National Diabetes fact sheet: http://apps.nccd.cdc.gov/DDTSTRS/FactSheet.aspx and http://www.cdc.gov/media/releases/2011/p0126_diabetes.html.

7. Haines, L., Chong, Wan K., Lynn, R., Barrett, T. G., Shield, J. P. H. "Rising incidence of type 2 diabetes in children in the United Kingdom." *Diabetes Care*, 30:1097–1101, 2007. http://www.cdc.gov/diabetes/projects/vda2.htm.

8. http://www.cdc.gov/obesity/data/trends.html.

9. Source: http://www.ahcpr.gov/CLINIC/uiovrvw.htm (accessed 1/24/08).

10. Vernikos, J. *The G-Connection: Harness Gravity and Reverse Aging.* Lincoln, Nebraska: iUniverse, Inc., 2004.

3

What Does Using Gravity Mean?

As was explained in chapters 1 and 2, research at NASA and other places has dramatically expanded our understanding of how gravity affects and interacts with the human body, and we went over how this research connects with the health epidemic afflicting most of the developed world. Although space flight research began more than 50 years ago, there is still much we don't know about how gravity affects our bodies. For example, we do not yet know all of the ways our body senses gravity and what all the various characteristics of gravity are. However, we *do* know gravity pulls down to the center of the earth, and it exerts its maximum effect when we stand up. We also know that sitting largely counteracts the beneficial effects of gravity.

Here in Chapter 3, I will share with you four lines of fascinating research that will help you better understand how to fight Gravity Deprivation Syndrome. If you really wish to, you can go ahead and start the Action Plan detailed in Part Two of this book. But the scientist in me urges you to continue reading, because the better you understand the science underlying the solution to GDS, the better your chances of faithfully adopting the G-habits that will lead you to live a long and healthy life.

CLUES FROM FOUR LINES OF RESEARCH

UNDOING THE EFFECTS OF STAYING IN BED

My own research into the effects of gravity deprivation with healthy human volunteers[1] led to this question: If one lies in bed continuously, what is the minimum amount of time per day one must spend upright—or walking upright at the mild pace of three miles per hour—to completely prevent Gravity Deprivation Syndrome, which continuous bed rest induces? We've learned that as little as four days in bed is sufficient to result in a reliably measurable case of GDS. In fact, orthostatic hypotension—fainting upon standing up—and a measurable reduction in blood volume are evident within 24 hours; so is an increased loss of calcium in the urine. Markers of bone loss can be detected in as little as three to four days, and aerobic fitness can decrease by as much as 25 percent within that same time frame. Changes happen very quickly when we thwart the helpful effects of gravity.

So, to find the minimum amount of time that must be spent upright, we had our subjects get up for 15 minutes, either every hour on the hour or every two hours, for a total of 16 to 8 times per day. Each subject went through all of the experimental conditions, and each was given a month between exposures to recover. In this way they served as their own controls. They stayed in bed and, for the "getting up" requirement, either simply stood by the bed or walked on a treadmill at a gentle pace. You would have guessed that walking would have been more effective. Much to my surprise, standing without exercise was more effective in the

---

BEWARE OF BEING TOO COMFORTABLE

Most people are more likely to sink into a comfortable chair when watching TV than in a straight-backed chair with no armrests. Is an armchair any worse than a straight-back or rocking chair? If you are less than comfortable when sitting, chances are you will fidget, change position, and probably get up more often without even realizing why. And that's good! Another form of discomfort that might work for you is not turning on the air-conditioner or setting it at a warmer temperature in the summer and cooler in the winter.

And is the TV the cause of today's sedentary society? The right study has not yet been carried to compare the effects of sitting with and without TV. Is sitting watching TV any worse than sitting taking a nap or sitting reading a book for the same length of time? Brain MRI studies would probably yield the answer right away. Chances are that different brain regions would be activated in each of the three scenarios—napping being a physiological consequence of sitting or lying down, reading likely stimulating imagination and creativity, and, with rare exceptions, TV acting as a pacifier.

---

regulation of blood pressure and the restoration of blood volume. When I thought about it, though, it made sense that standing without exercise required the cardiovascular system to pump blood up to the head unaided by contracting leg muscles. In fact, the longer one stands, the lesser the stimulation of the blood vessel walls, because when we stand still for very long our leg muscles start to quiver and contract to keep us upright. Thus, the shorter but more frequent changes in posture, the greater the benefit to the regulation of blood pressure.

Standing up often is what matters, not how long you remain standing. Every time you stand up, the body initiates a shift in fluids, volume, and hormones, and causes muscle contractions to occur; and almost every nerve in the body is stimulated. If you stand up 16 times a day for two minutes, the body would read that as 16 stimuli, whereas if you stood once and remained standing for 32 minutes, it would see that as one stimulus.

For the bed-bound volunteers in our study, as little as eight sessions of walking at three miles/hour for a total of two hours was plenty to prevent the loss of calcium, the appearance of bone-loss markers, and the decrease in aerobic stamina (max VO^2, a measure of aerobic capacity). We know from previous bed-rest studies that bicycling on a horizontal ergometer for as little as 30 minutes a day, even without getting out of bed, was enough to maintain stamina. Since we did not test shorter periods, it is probable that much less time walking on the treadmill for each bout would have been adequate. As muscles contract, they pull bone in every which way, even at the low speeds we used, as long as the subjects are upright or changing posture frequently.

At seminars, I like to ask my audiences how much and how often they exercise. Like me, they have been indoctrinated with the idea that the more exercise you do the better. Their answers range from three to five times a week and from 30 minutes to one hour a day. My question then is, "What do you do the other 23 hours? Well, given seven to eight hours of sleep, what do you do the other 15 to 16 hours?" This is invariably greeted by nervous giggles. I can just hear what they are thinking! "She is going to tell us the same old thing: Exercise more!" After all, people exercise to stay fit.

Exercise is effective in controlling obesity and Type 2 diabetes. It works by metabolizing fat calories that accumulate through the diet and it regulates insulin, free fatty acids, and triglyceride production by controlling sugar in the bloodstream. This implies that the more you work—the more strenuous and the more extended the exercise—the more fat would be metabolized. It can be difficult to convey to people that I am not talking about getting more exercise—I'm talking about a different *kind* of exertion. I am referring to the multitude of small, low-intensity movements we make throughout the day as we go about the business of living—movements that are related to using gravity. These are movements that *occur naturally throughout the day* when you're doing activities other than sitting. And yet these simple movements—these G-habits—are the key to health!

STABILIZERS, MOBILIZERS, AND THE METABOLIC BASIS OF USING GRAVITY

The second line of research came from observing nature and its relationship to physical therapy.[2] Have you ever wondered how migratory birds fly or fish swim, or how some mammals cover long distances, making optimum use of their energy without apparent fatigue? Dorothee Debuse and George Korfmacher at the University of Northumbria, United Kingdom, point out that animals use for these purposes a type of muscle that humans have as well, although our modern sedentary lifestyle has allowed it to weaken. Skeletal muscles can be categorized into two broad categories, depending on their structure and the way they work. Broadly speaking, the postural muscles, also referred to as slow or red muscles, whose primary function is to maintain the body's posture, are commonly known as "stabilizers"; those that move the body are "mobilizers."

Mobilizers, which are the muscles targeted in our traditional gym or training exercise routines, are capable of producing great force when they contract, although they are not able to do work for a long period of time because they quickly fatigue.

Stabilizers become weaker faster when they no longer have to work against gravity. In fact, the make-up of these muscle is such that they do best when they work for long periods of time without switching off. They can produce only low forces of contraction often with no obvious movement. Think of the deep muscles along your spine that keep you upright. If they did not work you would tilt forward. The back of your neck muscles support your head. If they are weakened your head would tip forward, which could be lethal.

SITTING IS NOT GOOD FOR MEN

There are good reasons why sitting contributes to erectile dysfunction (ED) and none why it should not. To listen to TV ads, you would have to believe that ED is yet another of our modern-day epidemics. Does it occur more than impotence ever did? Has it just come out of the closet, or is it just another example of the old and lucrative market for male enhancement? In ancient Egypt they chewed nutmeg—and still do. Today, Viagra is a household ingredient on the spice rack.

Testosterone levels are reduced in space and by lying in bed continuously, and should be with prolonged sitting. The same is true for the endothelium, the lining of the smooth muscle of blood vessels. The penis is a spongy tissue filled with blood vessels. An erection occurs when the endothelium is stimulated and the vessels relax and fill up with blood. That is how Viagra works. Furthermore, sitting occludes the blood circulation to the genital area, especially if one is overweight or obese. Anything that limits the amount of blood in the penis determines the extent of the erection. Men, sitting is not good for you and a short burst of exercise is not the answer.

Stabilizers, *the muscles least used in your gym exercises*, rely on low and sustained effort, less than 30 percent of a maximum voluntary contraction, and may or may not result in movement. Such energy efficiency depends on larger numbers of healthy mitochondria, the energy machines inside cells. Under conditions of reduced gravity use, such as space travel, inactivity, Type-2 diabetes, or aging, weaker muscle has fewer and smaller functional mitochondria. This results in disturbed oxidative metabolism, producing damaging oxygen peroxides, resistance to insulin, accumulation of fatty triglycerides inside the muscle, and a reduced protection by antioxidants. Loading up on antioxidant pills is a poor solution. However, Donal O'Gorman at Dublin City University, Ireland, points out that a simple correction of this dysfunction in stabilizer muscle cells would involve activities that use gravity in a manner that targets gene expression of mitochondrial and fatty acid oxidation processes to enrich mitochondria, increase oxidative capacity, and resistance to fatigue.[3]

What does all this mean? Why discuss insulin, diabetes, and obesity? As I'm sure it is clear by now, inactivity—too much sitting—makes you sick, and the standard exercise you are getting in the gym will not get to

you healthy. Next time you reach for that electric cart
or the golf course, give an extra thought to your stabi-
t make it possible for you to hang on to your indepen-
r your legs to carry you, and for you to stand up and
or neck pain.

IVITY THERMOGENESIS (NEAT)

About nine years ago, James Levine an exercise physiologist at the
Mayo Clinic in Rochester, Minnesota, coined the term non-exercise ther-
mogenic activity (NEAT).[4] His concept of NEAT sounded much like what
I had been discovering in my space and gravity-related research.

NEAT is a *much greater* component of your body's total energy expenditure throughout a typical day than are structured high-intensity exercises such as walking, running, bicycling, or working out in a gym. NEAT is
defined as the small, brief, yet frequent muscular movements one makes
throughout the day, of which changing position is the most effective:
standing, sitting, lying down, bending over to pick up something, squatting, stretching upward to take something off a shelf, getting dressed and
undressed, playing a musical instrument, and stirring a pot; even movements as small as crossing and uncrossing one's legs, waving one's hands
while talking, and fidgeting are helpful. It is these types of small movements and activities that do not happen enough when a person is habitually inactive. Whenever we move around, calories we have consumed
are converted into energy by contracting muscles and are measured as
generated heat—thermogenesis—the "T" of the "NEAT" acronym. Thus,
people who move around a lot all day, even if they don't go to the gym or
engage in intense exercise, burn up many more calories than people who
are sedentary. They even expend more calories than those who do go to
the gym, but then spend the rest of their day sitting around. Not surprisingly, the research on NEAT has shown a connection between the lack of
NEAT and obesity and metabolic diseases, like diabetes.

At the University of Missouri, Marc Hamilton and his group took this
research to the next stage by demonstrating that structured exercise and
NEAT act through different mechanisms and on different muscle fibers.[5]
Whereas it has been known for a long time[6] that both Type I and Type
II muscles respond to an intense bout of exercise with an increase in the
muscle cells' oxygen burning mitochondria, only the red, oxidative slow
Type II muscle fibers—the stabilizers—respond to non-exercise or natural
physical activities distributed intermittently throughout the day.

A critical finding particularly relevant to modern people is that inactivity that reduces or eliminates small, frequent movements interferes with sugar and fat metabolism. Deprived of the daily challenge of gravity, the metabolism of both astronauts in space and volunteers in bed is changed, with fat accumulating to replace muscle used to provide sufficient energy for the body. The oxidation of fatty acids is reduced, as are enzymes needed for fatty acid metabolism, indicating a decreased capacity to use fats for energy. Whether in bed or in space, insulin levels increase in the blood. High density lipoproteins (HDL; "good" cholesterol) decrease, whereas low density lipoproteins (LDL; "bad" cholesterol) increase.[7] Muscle rapidly becomes resistant to insulin within three days of bedrest[8], and probably earlier, given that the condition developed within one day of hind-limb inactivity in mice.[9] In Hamilton's inactivity studies, the enzyme lipoprotein lipase, needed to break down triglycerides and normally triggered by *anaerobic activity*—not requiring oxygen—is decreased and fat deposits accumulate in the abdomen and move in to replace lost muscle.

Increased levels of insulin are known to facilitate not only the transport of glucose into muscle, but also of cholesterol and fat into the cells of the arterial walls, stimulating the synthesis of cholesterol and fat in the arterial lining.[10] Gerald Reaven at Stanford University[11] and Robert Stout and John Valance-Owen at Queen's University, Belfast,[12] proposed that the increase in insulin and insulin resistance after a high carbohydrate meal lead to atherosclerosis. It stands to reason that similar changes in insulin levels and resistance after inactivity, together with reduced breakdown of triglycerides enabled by the activity of lipoprotein lipase, would be expected to lead to greater risk of atherosclerosis, as well.

Sure enough, more recent evidence points to structural damage in the form of stiffening of the heart and blood vessels resulting from a sedentary lifestyle. This stiffening is now believed to have a metabolic basis and is not merely an inevitable consequence of aging. These conditions can be prevented through exercise. Too much sitting leads to what has become known as "lipotoxicity," the accumulation of abnormal metabolites—such as triglycerides, the end-products of collagen—and advanced glycation products combining to form complex cross-links. These collagen cross-links are considered the cause of stiffening of the heart and blood vessels with age or a sedentary lfestyle.[13]

The common denominator of NEAT with what counteracts the effects of space and bedrest is that it requires upright posture to work, an obvious sign that *gravity* is involved. In fact, the requirement is for frequent postural change.[14] Sound familiar? You can see how easily NEAT principles apply to the simple, natural, everyday activities we've been discussing.

Hamilton's summary of effective non-exercise physical activity is that it primarily involves hundreds of movements per day while standing. This may be leisure or non-leisure activity, but the activity needs to occur frequently throughout the day, seven days a week, 365 days a year. *The intensity and duration of each bout of non-exercise activity does not have to be high.* These recommendations are identical to those of the gravity-using activities prescribed in this book, with the distinct difference that by considering the choice of activities from a gravity-using point of view, rather than only an inactivity perspective, a broader range of effective options becomes available. As a result, the key features that arise are low-intensity, frequent, alternating movements that use gravity to load the body, targeting the stabilizer posture muscles and providing a sense of direction for balance and coordination.

What is surprising is that the pivotal role of gravity in this metabolic shift has been known since the late 50s/early 60s through the pioneering work of Milt Smith and his students at the University of California, Davis, where the first research centrifuge was constructed. While using this machine, mice, rats, dogs, rabbits, chickens, and primates not only develop strong bones and muscles, but also have higher metabolic rates, higher oxygen consumption, their muscles take up more glucose and they lose essentially all spare fat living at 2G—spinning at two times earth's gravity—even though they are less active and eat more than they would living at 1G.[15]

The dramatic decrease in non-exercise activities in women that has occurred in recent years was brought to light in a survey of 2000 mothers, half of whom gave birth in the 1970s and half in the late 1990s/early 2000s.[16] According to this study, today's mothers do only half as much housework as the 1970s mothers did. Longer office hours and better cleaning machines and products were thought responsible for this finding. 10,000 steps per day is a popular recommended target of activity, yet most people in developed countries struggle to achieve that target. The state of Colorado has the lowest recorded level of obesity in the United States, but a 2005 study found the average Colorado man and woman walk only 6,700 and 6,400 steps respectively.[17] In contrast, a study of the

Amish (who do not drive cars, do not have electricity, and therefore do a great deal of manual labor, and for whom obesity is unknown) found that Amish men walked an average of 18,000 steps per day as compared to 14,000 steps per day for Amish women.[18]

MECHANICAL SIGNALS

The fourth and final line of research I want to share with you comes from an entirely different perspective. Clinton Rubin at the State University of New York (SUNY) at Stony Brook has been trying to find out why bone is lost through inactivity and as we age. In people who have the misfortune to suffer from osteoporosis, bones do not merely become thinner, they begin to look more like Swiss cheese as they lose their density. These osteoporotic holes in bone become filled with fat, as does the bone marrow. Based on the principle that exercise involves both metabolic (chemical) and mechanical (anything that pushes, pulls, or distorts) signals, Rubin and his team started playing with mechanical signals. The results were surprising. It turns out that bone density increases in response to short daily exposures to high frequency, mechanical signals (0.3G, where 1G is the Earth's gravitational pull) that are about three orders of magnitude *below* those induced by exercise and well below those that would arise even during walking or by the commercial weight loss vibrating machines. Contrary to current theory, Rubin claims that large signals, such as those created by a foot hitting a pavement, are not the best signal for bone. Instead, bone responds to signals that "are more like buzzing than pounding."

Rubin and his co-workers tested a menagerie of rats, mice, turkeys, sheep, and humans standing or sitting on his mechanically-induced vertically vibrating platform. They theorize that standing for 10–20 minutes on this platform, whose low level of vibrations are barely perceptible and which generates only 0.2–0.3G, "tricks" the body into thinking it is receiving a load-bearing strain, making the bones get stiffer and stronger. Rubin arrived at this approach by calculating that the kind of strain muscles continuously place on long bones while a person is sitting or standing is close to the oscillations provided by vertical (up and down) vibrations, and are not only important in augmenting bone mass, but also muscle performance. In fact, he favors the interpretation that the beneficial action on bone is mediated by muscle—that is, it acts first on muscle, which then stimulates bone as it pulls and tugs at it with each small contraction. Studies conducted with post-menopausal women standing on

> ### Shivering is NEAT
>
> At first glance, there would appear to be no obvious relationship between NEAT type of activities and this low-intensity, high-frequency vibration treatment. However, there are physiological thermogenic responses that are within the range of intensity and frequency of Rubin's vibration. We call it shivering! Exposed to severe cold, our body's defense is to raise body temperature through a series of low-intensity, high-frequency muscle contractions. Floris Wuyts at the University of Antwerp takes a calculated guess that the basic frequency of shivering may be around 5Hz with harmonics up to 30Hz.[20] Another example is that of restless people. Have you noticed that they tend to be thin? As their legs twitch at a high frequency, they are burning calories and producing energy as heat. Children stomp their feet and clap their hands, as we do, to warm themselves up—a wonderful NEAT activity.

this vibrating platform have also demonstrated positive results in preventing the bone loss that typically develops at that time of life.

Since bone, muscle, and fat cells all share a common stem cell derived from bone marrow, Rubin and his team studied the effect of these low-magnitude mechanical signals on fat cells in mice. Not unlike centrifuged animals living at 2G, who lose body fat while eating more food, mice that stood on the platform became thinner in spite of eating as much as those that did not use the platform—they therefore must have been burning more calories. Over a 15-week period of daily treatment, the team observed a 27 percent decrease in fat cell production, as well as a reduction in key risk factors associated with the onset of type-2 diabetes, such as triglycerides and free fatty acids.[19] Though one would not expect to maintain fitness, muscle mass, and strength on this low-intensity, high-frequency type of vibration regime, the results of such studies have not yet been reported. This is a hot new field as more researchers are exploring how this form of vibration works. For instance, an exciting new finding is that it stimulates an increase in the number of stem cells.

The question remains as to how the body perceives this particular mechanical stimulus and how it is translated into a bone response. Is loading, as when standing on the platform, necessary? Although one study with lower G signals was not encouraging, early observations in mice suggest that the effect persists, even when the vibrations are applied directly to the sole of the foot at 0.6G. If vibration indeed "tricks" the body into thinking it is bearing a load—which, after all, is a function of gravity— then the gravity signal may have similar characteristics to this type of mechanical signal and must be sensed by similar receptors. The sole of the foot is rich in gravity-sensitive receptors that sense position and remain silent in the absence of gravity in space and when one is bed-bound; they must be affected by prolonged sitting as well. What role does the nervous system play? Is the effect on bone local? Would this treatment benefit a paraplegic with spinal cord injury, a stroke patient, or someone with cerebral palsy? Does vibration, frequent standing, or habitual frequent, low-intensity activity throughout the day stretch the skin in areas like the feet and stimulate joints rich in gravity sensors? Is the response localized to the legs? There is much that remains to be discovered.

From birth, gravity guides our development. As body weight and mass increase, muscle, bone and other structures adapt and strengthen their size to meet mechanical demands. As we decrease this demand by increased sitting or reduced movement with age or habit, the opposite results—fat deposits accumulate, sugar eaten cannot be turned into energy, muscles waste and bones shrivel, and the heart, blood vessels, and joints stiffen and ache.

Repair is possible. When, through activity and exercise, the body moves, vibrates, stretches, and tenses against the force of gravity, these negative body changes become preventable. New nerve cells and connections grow and brain maps controlling balance and movement develop once more.[21]

INSTANT SLIM!

When my son was seven years old, I took him to a new pediatrician who suggested we cut back on what he ate because his weight was slightly above the range for his age. George replied: "If I were taller, I would be thinner!" Even as an adult, you can demonstrate the value of standing taller by consulting one of the many body mass index charts available on the Internet. Consider that many of us habitually go around in a semi-slouched posture that reduces our height by ½–1 inch. Say your height is 5'8" when you stand straight, but only 5'7" when you stand in your everyday "relaxed" posture. Look at a BMI chart and see how much difference that inch makes in your BMI! Without losing an ounce, if you stand up to your full 5'8," you will reduce your BMI—you actually will be slimmer.

Measuring Your Gravity Fitness

I hope by this point I have convinced you of the benefits of increasing your G-use and that you are more likely to find the solution to lifelong health in your home or your yoga class than in the gym. But, before you start the Action Plan in Chapter 4 and begin to make deliberate changes in your activity habits, try this simple test. Hold a five-pound weight straight out to your side while you stand or sit up straight and use a stopwatch to time how many seconds you can continue holding it without leaning or contorting yourself. Most men aged 45 to 65 are able to hold it up for two to three minutes, most women for 90 seconds. This gives you a rough idea of your *gravity fitness*. Refer back to this baseline gravity score as you make lifestyle changes and get healthier, and retake the test from time to time to measure your improvement.

Here is a chart showing the typical durations that a group of men and women of different age groups can keep holding a particular weight before muscle fatigue makes them drop their arm. The weight was held in the subjects' dominant arm, which was stretched out to the side at shoulder height.

	Age	3 lbs.	5 lbs.	8 lbs.	10 lbs.	15 lbs.
Men	25–40				60–120	30
	40–50		130–180		40–60	
	50–65		120–130	60–75	20–30	
	65–80	90–140	65–85			
Women	25–40		75–100	30–90		
	40–65		60–120			
	65–80	90–120	60–90			

Comparison of times in seconds that men and women of different ages can hold various weights (lbs,) with an outstretched dominant arm at shoulder height.

Tip: *Always remember that you are not measuring yourself up to what others can do, but how you improve against your own starting score.*

Another assessment you can make before you start is to have someone carefully measure your height, weight, and waist and hip measurements.

If you are really brave, try the "birthday suit" exercise: Look at yourself naked in a mirror from all sides. Where you see folds, make a mental note to eliminate them. Now pull yourself up straight, with shoulders pushed downward and tummy tightened. Note how many folds have disappeared—no diet, no exercise! That was not very difficult, was it? Hold that image. That is the way you can look all the time. Now, the next time you look at an advertisement of women who have lost weight on some magic diet, notice their posture in the "before" and "after" photos. In some, the only change you may detect is how they stand, but the impression given is that they look thinner.

Now stretch your arms up straight over your head, keeping your shoulders down. Presto! You look even thinner. Hold that image, too. That is the way you want to end up looking. As you get healthier, be sure to check your image often. It is a great way to get positive feedback!

You may also want to take the Health Assets Questionnaire (HAQ) assessment in the Appendix at this point. It will give you a fuller picture of your overall wellness and provide a benchmark against which to measure how much you are improving in various related health areas as you make better use of gravity. Note that the HAQ includes questions on sleep, stress and coping, eating habits, and weight. Together with physical activity, these form the foundation of a healthy body and mind.

But you may well ask, "What does gravity have to do with these factors?" Gravity ties in with everything. For example, have you considered that adequate sleep in a horizontal position provides energy and is just as important as the things you do upright? Sleeping upright or even sitting up, as you may have experienced during an overnight flight, is not nearly as refreshing as lying in bed. Pay attention to the quality of your sleep and make sure you get enough of it. It is now well documented that sleep deprivation contributes to obesity, stress, and poor performance.[22]

TAKING CHARGE OF YOUR GRAVITY USE

Now that you know where you stand on the gravity fitness scale and have established some baseline measurements, take a few minutes to think about your daily habits. What do you regularly do that uses gravity? For example, how many hours a week do you spend doing housework or yard work? Do you go out of your way to climb two or three flights of stairs instead of taking an elevator? When at work or when shopping, do you park a little distance from the building's entrance, even if closer spaces are available? Do you leave your car in one place and run a number of local errands on foot? Perhaps you are a city-dweller who walks everywhere, or perhaps you work at a job involving lots of lifting, bending, and changes in posture—if so, you are way ahead of the game.

Next, think when and where you have the opportunity to modify your habits. Instead of working through your coffee break or using the time to sit and have a snack, why not take a brisk walk around the building? If you pop into the grocery store to pick up just a few items, how about collecting your purchases in a handheld basket instead of wheeling a cart through the store? At the airport, would you be willing to walk alongside the people-mover, especially if you will be sitting for the next few hours on a long flight? Something as simple as standing up from your desk every 15 minutes, or even raising your arms above your head may seem insignificant, yet even these actions require some effort: Muscles are contracting, bones are stimulated. Your heart rate increases every time you get out of a chair. You use your sense of balance to straighten your posture as you rise. When you stand up, you are defying gravity by going in the opposite direction. Have you considered that you need to get blood to your head as well as your feet? Every little bit you do helps.

And, strangely enough, *attitude* may also be a significant factor. Remember that song, "Whistle While You Work?" How about thinking "strong" while you work? A recent study showed that even thinking of housework as exercise has benefits. Psychologist Ellen Langer at Harvard University[23] studied 84 women who worked as hotel housekeepers, cleaning rooms and changing sheets. Half the women were told that they should think of their work as exercise. They were even told how many calories they burned doing specific tasks: 40 calories for 15 minutes of changing linens, 50 calories for 15 minutes of vacuuming, 60 calories for 15 minutes of cleaning bathrooms. The other half were told nothing about any health benefits of their work. After four weeks, those told of the benefits had lowered their blood pressure by 10 percent and lost two pounds and 0.5 percent body fat on average. Dr. Langer concluded "the changes were a function of the change in mind-set alone." She added, "If you are just sitting on the couch and just telling yourself that you're exercising, you're not going to believe yourself and so there will be no change."

It's All about Good Habits

You now have assessed where you are and you are motivated to get moving. As you embark on your journey to healthfulness, always remember to listen to your body—it thrives on variation and new challenges. Try to eventually do all of the recommended activities in this book's Action Plan. As you progress, you may find the distribution of fat and muscle in your body will improve. You will regain lost height. Best of all, you will feel so much better and will have so much more energy.

If you are active and exercise regularly, or play some sport, or take a yoga class, *keep it up.* If you already have excellent posture and balance, good for you. *Do not change what already works!* As you develop your Action Plan in Chapter 4, focus on those activities that you no longer do, or work on new ones you had not thought of and add them to your repertoire. Play with your options. There is no set sequence—you are free to tailor your own individualized plan.

> **Tip:** *I find that I am more likely to stay active and keep up my good habits throughout the week if I take as little as one exercise class a week. I prefer something like yoga that is gravity-oriented and works on stretching, posture, and flexibility. But any kind of exercise class might do. However, going to the gym once a week, even if working with a personal trainer, does not count as a class. It is the group aspect that seems to do it for me. Social interaction and shared experience is good for the soul.*

Gravity-habits are good habits. A great way to take charge of your G-use and track your progress is to make your own gravity diary, and study it. Record how many hours a day you spend sitting. Too much sitting is bad for you! Knowing this, you might think that the solution would be to spend more time standing—but this is not so. Workers in the retail trade or others whose job includes six hours a day standing often suffer from varicose veins, as well as foot, hip, and knee joint problems. It is developing the G-habit of standing up often, changing your position relative to gravity, that is the most beneficial way of using gravity.

A simple pedometer measures the number of steps you take every day and is a great way to track your progress. Record the average number of steps you take for about three days in your diary. This gives you an overall measure of your current level of activity. Though steps may not register the gravity value from these moves, they do serve as a rough indicator of your overall activity level. Then, each week, retake this measurement for two successive days. Watch your record grow. In addition to recording how many steps you take, make note of how many times you stand up and the types of movements you make. Congratulate yourself on the beneficial habits you already have, then see what you can do to improve. It's all about gravity *habits*. As time goes on, your diary will reflect more and more the movements and actions you turn into habits—your "G-habits."

Even if others do not compliment you—but they will!—you will feel more confident as your G-use increases. Friends will say "you have changed your hairstyle" or "you have lost weight." But only you know why you've changed. How you appear to yourself when you go by a mirror, along with compliments from others, counts as progress. Now—let's get started!

Moving Habits Are Child's Play

The sitting epidemic is now spreading to children. Instead of playing hopscotch, chasing balls, and climbing trees, children exercise their thumbs playing GameBoy and texting their friends, or staring at the PC and TV screen. How can parents get their kids off their seat and back to health? Telling them to get up and go or signing them up for a sport is a sure way to produce a good result.

The best way is to develop healthy lifetime habits, not only for the children, but also for the parents, grandparents, or anyone else in their family environment. Children mimic, and they will tend to mimic the sloth in the family. If it takes periodic family conferences to get people moving, so be it. Moving will help everyone's health and vigor. Give the children the responsibility to get everyone moving. If you find it annoying or come up with excuses, think how they feel when you tell them what to do. Spend more family fun time outdoors, camping, biking, hiking, or ask them to help you weed or plant in the garden. Ask for their physical help, from opening a jar, reaching for something, or getting you a glass of water. Make physical achievement a thing of pride. You get the idea.

CHAPTER 3 NOTES

1. Vernikos, J., Ludwig, D. A., Ertl, A. C., Wade, C. E., Keil, L.C., O'Hara, D. "Effect of standing or walking on physiological changes induced by head down bed rest." *Aviat Space Env Med* 67:1069–1079, 1996.

2. Taylor, G., Thomas, A., Nudds, R. "Flying and swimming animals cruise at a strouhal number tuned for high power efficiency." *NATURE* 425:707–711, 2003.

3. O'Gorman, D. J. Personal communication, 2009; O'Gorman, D. J., Karlsson, H. K. R., McQuaid, S., Yousif, O., Rahman, Y., Gasparro, D., Glund, S., Chibalin, A.V ., Zierath, J. R., Nolan, J. J. "Exercise training increases insulin-stimulated glucose disposal and GLUT-4 protein content in patients with Type-2 diabetes." *Diabetologia* 49:2983–2992, 2008.

4. Levine, J. A., Schleusner, S. J., Jensen, M. D. "Energy expenditure of nonexercise activity." *Am J Clin Nutr* 72 (6):1451–1454, 2000; see also Levine, J. A., Lanningham-Foster, L. M., McCrady, S. K., Krizan, A. C., Olson, L. R., Kane, P. H., Jensen, M. D., Clark, M. M., Levine, J. A., Vander Weg, M. W., Hill, J. O., Klesges, R. C. "Non-exercise activity thermogenesis: the crouching tiger hidden dragon of societal weight gain." *Arterioscl Thromb Vasc Biol* 26(4):729–736, 2006.

5. Hamilton, M. T., Hamilton, D. G., Zderic, T. W. "The role of low energy expenditure and sitting on obesity, metabolic syndrome, type 2 diabetes, and cardiovascular disease." *Diabetes* 56(11):2655–2667, 2007.

6. Winder, W. W., Baldwin, K. M., Holloszy, J. O. "Enzymes involved in ketone utilization in different types of muscle: adaptation to exercise." *Eur J Biochem* 47: 461-467, 1974.

7. Nicogossian, A. E., Huntoon, C. L., Poole, S. L. *Space Physiology and Medicine*. Philadelphia: Lea and Febiger, 1994.

8. Lipman, R. I., Raskin, P., Love, T., Triebwasser, J., Lecocq, F. R., Schnure, J. J. "Glucose intolerance during decreased physical activity in man." *Diabetes* 21:101–107, 1972.

9. Seider, M. J., Nicholson, W. F., Booth, F. W. "Insulin resistance for glucose metabolism in disused soleus muscle of mice." *Am.J.Physiol.* 242:E12–E18, 1982.

10. Stout, R. "Insulin stimulation of cholesterol synthesis by arterial tissue." *Lancet* 294(7618):467–468, 1969.

11. Reaven, G. M. Banting Lecture 1988: "Role of insulin resistance in human disease.", *Diabetes* 37(12):1595–1607, 1988.

12. Stout, R., Valance-Owen, J. "Insulin and Atheroma." *Lancet* 293(7605):1078–1080, 1969.

13. Prasad, A., Levine, B. D. *Aging and Diastolic Heart Failure*, A Klein and M Garcia Eds. GW Medical Publishing, St.Louis, Chapter 30: pp385–400, 2008.

14. Levine, J. A., Lanningham-Foster, L. M., McCrady, S. K., Krizan, A. C., Olson, L. R., Kane, P. H., Jensen, M. D., Clark, M. M. "Interindividual variation in posture allocation: possible role in human obesity." *Science* 307:584–586, 2005.

15. Evans, J. W., Smith, A. H., Boda, J. M. "Fat metabolism and chronic acceleration." *Amer. J. Physiol.* 216:1468–1471, 1969.

16. Andrews, Emily, *Daily Mail*, October 11, 2007.

17. Wyatt, H. R., Peters, J. C., Reed, G. W., Barry, M., Hill, J. O. "A Colorado statewide survey of walking and its relation to excessive weight." *Med Sci Sports Exerc* 37:724–730, 2005.

18. Bassett, D. R., Schneider, P. L., Huntington, G. E. "Physical Activity in an Old Order Amish Community." *Med Sci Sports Exerc* 36:79–85, 2004.

19. Rubin, C. T., Capilla, E., Luu, Y. K., Busa, B., Crawford, H., Nolan, D. J., Mittal, V., Rosen, C. J., Pessin, J. E., Judex, S. "Adipogenesis is inhibited by brief, daily exposure to high frequency, extremely low-magnitude mechanical signals." *PNAS* (6 Nov) 104(45):17879–17884, 2007.

20. Floris L Wuyts, Director, Antwerp Research Center for Equilibrium and Aerospace, Dept of Physics, U of Antwerp, Belgium. Personal communication, 2008.

21. Langer, E. *Counterclockwise: Mindful Health and the Power of Possibility*. Ballantine Books, 2009.

22. Laposky, A. D., Bass, J., Kohsaka, A., Turek, F. W. "Sleep and circadian rhythms: Key components in the regulation of energy metabolism." *FEBS Letters*, 582(1):142–151, 2008.

23. Langer, E. *Counterclockwise: Mindful Health and the Power of Possibility*. Ballantine Books, 2009.

PART TWO:

PUTTING GRAVITY TO WORK FOR LIFELONG HEALTH

4

Your Action Plan

We've all heard of exercise and diet plans that promise to change our lives for the better in just 30 days. And most of us have seen these plans fail, either for ourselves or others, or at best bring initial results that soon taper off. These plans are usually hard to keep up because they don't fit well into our lives. The good news is that when it comes to gravity and the benefits it brings you don't have to disrupt your life or schedule. There are unlimited opportunities for fitness all around us. The key to success lies in increasing the amount of natural, habitual physical activity we engage in throughout the day, each and every day of our lives; in other words, we must engage in frequent movement, a sort of perpetual motion. But how do we do this?

TURN ALL DAY, NATURAL NON-EXERCISE ACTIVITIES INTO G-HABITS

Developing a varied set of habitual *non-exercise* movements is the most important thing you can do. Even if you do exercise regularly at the gym, pay attention to your habits when you are not exercising, for they benefit your body in a very different way. If your life and work are such that you cannot get away to exercise, you do not enjoy playing a sport, and you spend much of your day sitting in an office or a car, all is not lost. This is all the more reason why you will derive great benefits from restoring gravity habits—G-habits—back into your life. You had these habits as a growing child, so it's simply a question of getting them back.

Healthy seniors seem to have benefited from G-habits, perhaps because they retain those activities that target the stabilizer muscle system.

Think of your grandmother or aunt who would never ignore a speck of lint on the floor, but quickly bent over to pick it up. "She has always hated exercise," says Elsa, describing her vigorous, 92-year-old mother. "But she is always getting out of her chair to get something from the kitchen, straighten the afghan on the sofa, or putter with her plants. Even while riding in the car, she never sits still; she's always fidgeting with her hair or her purse or the seat belt. In an everyday conversation, she's the type who couldn't talk if she didn't wave her hands."

> **Tip:** *Exercise is not a substitute for activities that come naturally throughout the day, 365 days a year, for the rest of your life.*

Developing good G-habits takes time. Do not expect overnight results. Eight to 12 weeks is a reasonable time frame to cement new G-habits into your daily ritual, although you'll start noticing the good results from these habits much sooner than that. Do not try to work on too many new habits at the same time. Work incrementally. This is crucial to lifelong success because the object is to acquire, restore, or rediscover lifelong habits. Such habits must be realistic and mesh with your particular lifestyle. Only when an activity becomes a habit will it become part of your daily life, rather than a chore that must be remembered, like medicine that must be taken.

For optimal effectiveness, the intensity of your G-habits should be low. Gentle movements that challenge gravity's direction and acceleration, and all strength moves as well, specifically work on developing those precious maps in the brain that control our balance and coordination. This gentle approach also strengthens the all-important stabilizers in your body which, as we discussed earlier in the book, are traditionally neglected by conventional exercise regimens, which focus on mobilizers. For many people, this focus on mobilizer exercise has resulted in chronic pain, mostly in the back. When stabilizers atrophy, as they frequently do in our modern sedentary lifestyle, mobilizers cannot function properly because they lack a firm base from which to work. The consequence of this is instability of segments of the body, distorting the movement and causing lower back pain or even falls. Among the styles of exercise we typically see today, yoga and tai chi—which, you will note, are ancient forms of activity—are the exceptions, as they target mainly stabilizers. Maintaining fitness of stabilizers through continuous low-intensity activities forms the foundation of a healthy, active body. Performing repetitive, sustained, low-intensity activities throughout the day is nature's way of not allowing the stabilizer system to weaken.

Some activities are more gravity-effective than others. For example, every time you stand up from a sitting position, you are moving your entire upper body against gravity. You cannot measure a movement like this with a pedometer (unfortunately, the perfect gravity-activity monitoring device, combining measurement of steps taken, mechanical stimulation, and acceleration, has not yet been developed). Nevertheless, it's a great idea to increase your gravity awareness by tracking your activities, which helps you quantify your progress as habits become second nature. Why not consciously count how many times a day you stand up? Then, set a target and work up to it. Make it fun by counting down from your target number like a space rocket liftoff—36, 35, 34.... You will discover it takes at least a week or two to strengthen new G-habits to the point where repetitions no longer need to be counted and the activity has been seamlessly integrated into your life.

There is no end to the number of new habits you could explore and develop. Some, like stretching and standing up, you must do every day. Others, like housecleaning, gardening, or sports activities will be done less often. Try to introduce new habits on a frequent basis. If you get stuck about wondering what else you can do, be a child again. Play. Have fun! Take stock in how much better you look and feel so that you reach the point, just as with brushing your teeth, where you cannot conceive of life without the healthful G-habits that have become an enjoyable part of your daily routine.

If you are like me, you have a limited amount of time and energy available to devote to structured exercise in the gym, particularly if you include travel time, time for dressing and undressing, showering, and the increased laundry produced by sweaty exercise attire. You need something you can live with for the rest of your life, without injuries or calculators. You want your activities and exercise to be targeted and efficient, with a maximal response for minimal effort. You need variety, practical choices, measurable success, and rewards. I designed the G-habits Action Plan that follows so that you can be inventive and can pick, choose, and tailor from the list of activities those that best suit your lifestyle.

Here are some comparative estimates of G value that may be generated from various activities, conditions or devices. Gz means that G is pulling in the head-to-toe direction; Gx is pulling across the chest. Most of these are estimates.

Activity	G-Value
Standing on Earth	1Gz
Standing on Mars	0.33Gz
Standing on the Moon	0.16Gz
Lying down on Earth	0Gz / 1Gx
Sitting on Earth	< 1Gz
Stand up from Lying down	0 to 1Gz
Walking	1.3–1.5Gz
Standing on C. Rubin's Vibrating Plate	1.2–1.3Gz (1G for standing +0.2–0.3Gz g-strain)
Running	1.6–2.3Gz
Roller Coaster	2 to 2.3Gz
Trampoline	Up to 4.5Gz
Jumping	2.5 to 6Gz
Centrifuge (horizontal on short-arm centrifuge)	0 to 2.5Gz
Centrifuge (swing-out seat on long arm)	<1 to 8Gz

Eight Fundamentals of G-Effective Activity

Before you begin your action plan, let me share some recommendations about how to use natural activities most effectively so that you can make the best investment of your precious time and energy.

1. Which One? What to Choose?

The short answer is "All": posture and balance challenges for your stabilizer muscles and your brain, stretching movements for flexibility, strength-building movements for your mobilizer muscles, as well as aerobic intensity for improving your stamina and cardiovascular fitness.

2. How Long?

The short answer is "All Day." That is, all-day G-*habits*, which is not the same thing as all-day exercise. If you are already working out in a gym, continue your gym routine until you have gradually introduced a full complement of G-habits in addition to your other usual daily activities—then decide whether to cut down on exercise. If you are starting from scratch, begin by increasing your everyday activity with G-habits. Estimate and note the number of hours you spend sitting or lying down during the day. Aim to spend less time sitting still or slouched.

3. How Much?

This is not an easy question to answer, because G-habits are so varied that they don't lend themselves to easy measurement. A pedometer is a useful general guide for estimating overall activity, but is not reliable as a gravity or habit indicator. Simply estimating the number of hours you spend each day engaged in activities versus sitting may be a better indicator. (By the way, driving counts as sitting.) Habits offering you a range of high- and low-intensity activity are what you need to keep your body tuned.

4. Intermittent—Alternate Fast and Slow

Habits are activities we do intermittently throughout the day. This is a very important reason why G-habits are so beneficial. For example, if you stand up once and sit right back down, your body sees this as the same single stimulus as if you remain standing for 30 minutes. And if you stand up 15 times over the course of, say, one hour, your body sees it as 15 new stimuli and responds every time you stand. Consequently, standing up 15 times throughout your day, allowing time to recover completely between stands, is more effective than standing and sitting 15 times in rapid succession. You may already be familiar with this concept from interval training in exercise—alternating slow and fast bursts of walking, running, cycling, or swimming, or in fact any exercise.

5. Intermittent—Alternate Hard and Easy

Some habitual natural activities that make good G-habits are more strenuous than others. Think of carrying a heavy bag of groceries up a flight of stairs, or setting up and climbing a 20-foot ladder to clean the gutters on a two-story house. These are much more strenuous than cooking a meal or making a bed. Alternating hard and gentler movements is a more effective approach than sustaining activity at the same level. If you do strength training exercise, you may have learned the benefit of doing a few very slow *maximum effort* repetitions, and then switching to a set of 10–12 repetitions with a lighter load.

6. ADD VARIETY

Always bear in mind that too little or too much of anything is not good. Variety in movement is extremely important. As with intermittent speed and intensity, the body becomes less responsive to the same repeating stimulus. That is a basic reason why turning all-day natural activities into habits is so crucial. Most people I know who go to a gym have a set exercise routine they follow daily. This may be fine for maintenance, but if you are looking for continued improvement, you should vary your routine, rather than concentrate on building greater intensity or duration. Make it a habit to build in variety; avoid doing exactly the same routine in the same order at the same time every day.

7. THINK GRAVITY—THINK DIRECTION

Remember that gravity pulls on your body from head to toe, so gravity's maximum effect is felt when you *are standing*. Whenever you have a choice, increase the benefit by doing your G-activities standing up. Similarly, if you do strength training, shoulder presses standing on one leg in which you hold a weight overhead increases the gravity effectiveness of the exercise, since both weight and balance are gravity dependent.

8. CLOSE YOUR EYES

Doing any activity or exercise with eyes shut enhances the influence of gravity and makes us realize how much we grow to depend on vision instead of our inner ear for balance. As a plus, if you are subject to motion sickness, you may find your next trip on a plane or boat less troublesome after you have gotten into the habit of moving your body and changing your posture with your eyes closed.

With these eight fundamentals in mind, you are ready to devise your action plan. When you incorporate G-habits into your life, you are moving toward the perpetual motion goal that will help you stay vigorous and independent.

G-Habits Action Plan

By **Star Rating** habits, activities, and exercises (like the star rating system for hotels and restaurants), I've indicated which are of the most benefit. And for those of you who are used to thinking in terms of calories burned, I also give you an estimate of the energy value of each move as total **calories burned** or calories per hour for a 120–140-pound person. If your weight is different, divide the calories burned for each activity by 130 and multiply by your body weight in pounds to get the calories you would burn. You will notice that calories do not always correlate with gravity-value star rating, but both are important for good health and fitness. Expressed as calories per minute or per hour, you would need to calculate the duration of each activity to estimate how many calories were burned. For instance, carrying bags of groceries to your car uses up the same number of calories/hour—180—as carrying a baby around in a sling or backpack, but you would likely spend only a few minutes carrying the groceries, whereas many new parents carry their baby for an hour or more at a time.

There are innumerable core habits we all do at one time or another, the most obvious being light housework like vacuuming (a ** rating), good for 200 calories an hour (cals/hr). More strenuous activities like raking and picking up leaves and shoveling snow (****) could be worth up to 350 cals/hour. Milder gardening, pruning, planting, weeding, and mowing (* to ****) could be worth 300–350 cals/hour; plus, they increase stamina and work long-neglected muscles. Less strenuous is a stand-up stimulus, such as getting a glass of water—still, this simple effort yields tremendous gravity value (****; 10–15 cals/hr). You might also carry a baby (***; 180 cals/hr), stir a large pot of Sophia Loren's pasta sauce recipe (**; 132 cals/hr), roll out cookie dough (**; 132 cals/hr), crack nuts (*; 100 cals/hr), or carry your grocery bags to the car (***; 15 cals/hr). You might take the garbage bin out (**; 18 cals/hr), paint a room (****; 270–350 cals/hr), scrub the bathtub (***; 160 cals/hr), paint your fence (****; 300–350 cals/hr), grow your own vegetables (**; 100–150 cals/hr), and get fit![1]

Here's an important tip: You can vary the activities in the following list by doing each move, such as standing up or sitting down, as slowly as you possibly can. This will make them harder to do, thereby yielding greater G-value. Remember: *Keep gravity in mind as you do these activities.* That should help you focus on what you're doing and remember why it is important to your health. Ready to start? Here we go!

Get back into the Stretching Habit *****

Muscles/ Joints/ Ligaments/ Tendons/ Bones/ Spine/ Neck/ Shoulders/ Feet (100 cals/hr)

We think of a child waking up with a good stretch, and we've all noticed that cats and dogs do the same thing. But many of us just stumble out of bed when the alarm goes off. As you age, or if you have stopped stretching at any age, your muscles tighten and the range of motion in your joints decreases. This can put a damper on active lifestyles and even hinder day-to-day, normal motions. Tasks that used to be simple, such as zipping up a dress or reaching for a jar on the top shelf, now become difficult. The AARP's driving course for seniors includes stretching exercises as a safety precaution. Many elderly drivers lose their range of neck motion to such a degree that they cannot rotate their head to look behind them when backing out of a parking space or driveway—the result is often an accident! A regular stretching or yoga program can help lengthen your muscles and make daily living activities easier.

> **Tip:** Do not bounce when you stretch, as this can put strain on tendons and joints. Extend the stretch as far as you can and hold it, continuing to breathe naturally. You may use a timer or a clock that displays seconds to time your stretches—30 seconds is good, 60 seconds is better.

Get back into that stretching habit. Even before you get out of bed, twirl your feet several times in each direction. Then do the same with your hands, and rotate your shoulders. Next, sit up and clasp your hands and stretch them straight up over your head, pushing your shoulders downward. Turn your hands inside out if you can, with palms facing the ceiling. Stand up and stretch some more (remember the "Bend and Stretch" song from *Romper Room*?). Take a few more minutes to lie down on the floor and repeat your stretch, pulling your feet and hands in opposite directions. Relax completely and repeat two or three times. Bring your knees up, hug them, and roll from side to side or in slight circles in each direction. It feels wonderful for your back. Roll over to your right side and with your left hand push yourself gently up, head coming up last so that you do not feel light-headed. Finally, before you stand up, come up on your hands and knees and arch your back like a cat. In the few minutes it takes to do these stretches, you've now worked out the body kinks you acquired during the night and you are all relaxed, ready to start your day.

Everyone can learn to stretch again, regardless of age or flexibility. Have you noticed that singers have very few wrinkles? It's because they stretch their facial muscles. Stretching the skin is just as important as stretching the joints and ligaments; they are all collagen and respond to the mechanical push and pull. Stretching should be a part of your daily routine, whether you exercise or not. In addition to stretching when you wake up in the morning, you can stretch while watching TV, working on the computer, getting ready for bed, or any time you feel some tightness creeping in. Stretch your arms often behind your seat while sitting at your desk. If you are doing strength training exercises, stretch between sets. It feels good and saves time from stretching at the end of the workout!

While it does not have to involve a huge time commitment, developing good stretching habits can end up giving you huge results! Here are just a few of the benefits you can expect from a regular habit of stretching:

- Reduced muscle tension
- Increased range of movement in the joints
- Improved muscular coordination
- Increased circulation of the blood to various parts of the body
- Increased energy levels (resulting from increased circulation)
- Stress relief
- Tighter skin

> **Tip:** *Whenever you are not sure about what to do next, think of that child in you and stretch.*

Stand Up: Sit Down *****

Blood Pressure Control/ Muscles/ Joints/ Bones (2 cals/min)

If you do nothing else from this book, this is the *single most important habit* you can acquire. The key to independence in old age is being able to stand up. It's no more complicated than that. Start practicing now so you will be able to stand up and sit down without help for as long as you live.

Do this exercise correctly to get the most out of it. From a using-gravity perspective, standing up is excellent, especially if you raise your weight out of the chair *slowly* and repeat it many times throughout the day. If you stand up quickly the same number of times, but in a short period, it is an aerobic exercise—note how your heart beats faster and you pant.

Research indicates it would take at least 32 posture changes from sitting to standing and back again to maintain healthy blood pressure regulation. I know this for a fact from my studies with volunteers lying in bed continuously, 24 hours a day for four days. It took standing up from bed 16 times a day to prevent the tendency to faint when they got up. That means it took that many changes in posture to maintain the blood pressure that the sensors measured. It would take as many as 32+ times of standing from sitting, since that is a smaller change in the gravity stimulus than it is from lying down to standing. Consider 32 your lowest goal. More will not hurt you, though less may not produce the desired effect.

(a) On the Way Up you defy gravity. How do you get out of your chair? Do you lean on the arms of the chair? Do you lean on your knees? Create opportunities to get up often—for example, ask a neighbor to ring your doorbell and say hello as she goes by. Keep your mobile phone at a distance, or dock it so you have to get up to answer it. When watching TV, get your own drink. Drink plenty of water so that you must get up to use the bathroom often.

Aspire to stand up without leaning on anything. However, even if at first you do use furniture for support, you are strengthening the arms. Once standing up without support is mastered, do it very slowly to perfect it. Then try getting up from a low armchair or sofa without the help of the firm seat. That adds challenge to this habit.

(b) Getting Down is easy because gravity pulls you down. All you have to do is give in to it, and presto! you are back on your seat with a loud "plop." But that wastes this motion. To really benefit, you need to sit down

---

Tip: When I recommended frequent standing up at one of my talks, a man in the audience complained he could not do that because he worked all day with a computer. If he stood up too often, his boss would fire him. Asked whether he drank water, he replied, "Yes, of course. I have a bottle on my desk." "Put it on a shelf just far enough so that you have to stand up to reach it! It does double duty, keeping you toned and hydrated."

---

very slowly, resisting the pull of gravity all the way down—remember the mental image of a string pulling the top of your head toward the ceiling. Maintain good posture, and the more slowly you sit down, the more benefit your muscles get. That is a great leg strengthening exercise. Are you getting the idea? Slow is good.

(c) Squatting is a variation of sitting, but without the chair: Your knees are bent at an acute angle and your buttocks are near the floor. Watch a small child moving about and you will likely see a lot of effortless squatting—just think, when you were that age you did it, too. For some cultures, squatting is the normal seated position for adults and children alike, often preferred for eating and other seated activities; squatting is also practiced during childbirth. For everyone, it is the most efficient position for going to the bathroom, as it allows gravity to help the rectum expel waste. Holding a squat position strengthens the large thigh muscles. Standing up from a squat is an even greater gravity stimulus than getting up from a chair—but be careful the first few times you try it, as you might feel light-headed.

A bonus of standing up after squatting—and to a lesser extent after sitting—is that it sends blood up to your brain. Not too many other movements do that; your brain will thank you.

STAND TALL *****

BALANCE/ BACK AND NECK MUSCLES/ SPINE/ HEIGHT (2 CALS/MIN)

Remember that gravity pulls straight down, so standing tall makes you work upward against gravity. The straighter your posture, the more G-value, as you position your body in the optimal orientation to receive gravity's pull. Our head weighs about 15 pounds and sits on top of the spine. If the spine is not straight to support it and if the neck muscles are weak, the head will flop, as is the case with newborn babies (and with some frail elderly persons). The head is the only weight the upper spine carries. It serves to keep the bone density of the spine strong. Many of us tend to drop our head forward when we sit or walk. However, doing this reduces our spine's work against gravity, and so it weakens, can become frail, our back muscles hurt, and we lose height.

When you stand and sit, practice good posture, with a strong back, shoulders down, and back and abdominal muscles slightly flexed. Scrunching up your shoulders will put tension onto your neck muscles. To check your posture, stand with your back against a wall: Though your spine has a natural "s"-shaped curve, your lower back should be straight enough that you can't slip your hand in and out freely between your body and the wall.

> **Tip:** *My yoga teacher says, "Imagine a string pulling straight up from the top of your head." Raising your shoulders does no good, so keep them down and stretch your head upward toward the string. I once had a hairdresser who used to pull my hair when she washed it. It was torture. I would catch myself squirming up toward her to avoid the pain. You can do the same, without the hair-washing discomfort.*

STRETCH AT YOUR DESK ****

POSTURE/ SHOULDER BLADES/ LIFT CHEST/ TENSION RELIEF (1 CAL/MIN)

As you work at your desk, hold your head high away from your shoulders. Make sure you are not dropping it forward. Bend your left arm behind your back to grab the elbow of the right arm held straight downward beside you. You will immediately feel your shoulder blades come together, your shoulders move downward, and your chest rise. Hold as long as you can. Alternate arms. Repeat often. This stretch releases shoulder tension, as well as strengthening the good posture habit. Grasping your hands behind your back can also help you relieve the tension in your back.

Sitting in armchairs does no good to your posture because your elbows are raised and rest forward. I found an easy way to train the shoulder blades back is to sit with your hands resting high up on your thighs. Holding this position naturally presses the shoulder blades together.

Here is another easy variation as you work: Keeping both arms against your sides and bent at the elbow, move the elbows backward, bringing your shoulder blades together. Hold it. When you become good at it, you can work on your keyboard in this position. This stretch is also great on long flights or when waiting at traffic lights. If you make this move often while you work at your desk and while you sit at traffic lights holding your shoulders down, you will greatly reduce your risk of suffering from a stiff neck and shoulders.

Walk Tall *****

Posture/ Balance/ Spine/ Neck Muscles (150–350 cals/hr)

When you walk, remember that toddlers, as well as astronauts returning to Earth, walk with their legs far apart to keep from falling. Keep your sense of balance strong and move like a runway model by walking with your legs and feet close together. Aim to keep your gaze focused straight ahead rather than at your feet. This will help you walk taller and keep your spine strong.

A brisk walk in a park or other pleasant surroundings can be emotionally rewarding, too. If you take an hour to walk two miles, you will burn a good number of calories (144 to 168 calories for a 120- to 140-pound person, more if you're larger). On the other hand, a brisk or power walk of two miles in 40 minutes burns 192 to 222 calories, depending on your weight. If you want to burn twice as many calories for the same distance in the same time, try carrying a backpack. But whatever you do, be sure to walk tall! The emphasis is on moving briskly and with purpose. Why brisk? Think back to Chapter 3 and the value of intermittent, low-intensity, high-frequency movement. Walking is a series of intermittent steps, each one generating a vertical gravity stimulus by its impact. The faster you take those steps, the higher the frequency.

Former astronaut and U.S. Senator John Glenn makes a habit of power-walking two miles a day. And he works with weights three times a week. Power-walking is covering more ground in less time while swinging your arms outward at the same time. Glenn started doing this long before a recent study showed that gait speed—how fast you walk—helps you live longer.[2] The study concluded that the ideal for people over 65 was walking 2.25 miles in one hour every day. As I write this, John Glenn is 90 and still going strong. He must be doing something right!

The Stairs Option ***

Balance/ Coordination/ Muscle/ Bone/ Joints (8–10 cals/min)

Start off by taking the easy way up—elevator, escalator—and using the stairs going down. Going up stairs and going down stairs are two separate kinds of activities. Going down has a greater balance component; in addition, the impact loading with each step as you accelerate forward provides gravity stimulus to your legs, hips, and lower spine bones. Going up is more of an aerobic activity and builds stamina. It is also a form of weight training, as you pull your weight up each step. Going both up and down stairs are great exercises to strengthen muscles, but they work on different muscles, so you need to do both to strengthen both the front and back leg muscles—eccentric and concentric.

(a) Down—I am amazed at how early in life balance problems appear, especially in women. Ask young women in their 20s whether they need to look at their feet while going down the stairs and you will be surprised to find how many do. Many also hold onto the rail. In my personal poll of young receptionists, a quarter of them said they looked at their feet, and about a tenth did that and held onto the rail. What do you do? If you are unsteady on your feet, wait until you get stronger to try this, or start off by holding the rail. Put on a pair of low-heeled, comfortable shoes and test yourself. If you hold the rail, try to barely touch it until you acquire the confidence to do without it. Instead of keeping your eyes on the stairs all the time, try to look ahead a few steps at a time as you descend. If you find this difficult, build up to it by stepping on and off a low step stool while alternating feet. Once you master that, check the stairs again. Work on increasing the number of flights you're taking and on letting go of the rail. Your goal is to descend an entire flight without looking at your feet and without touching the rail. (I recommend you evaluate yourself using the scale in the book *Age-Defying Fitness*.)[3]

Many older persons avoid leaving their homes because they are afraid of falling when stepping up onto a bus, or even into an SUV-type vehicle. The step-stool exercise mentioned above can help them regain their confidence and independence by strengthening the necessary muscles and their sense of balance in the safety of their home.

(b) Up—Add going up stairs to coming down stairs. Climb stairs till you are just out of breath. Now let go of the rail and look straight ahead, not down at the stairs. Then increase the number of flights. If you don't have too many flights to climb, take every opportunity to choose the stairs rather than the easier method.

> **Tip:** *Did you know that going down stairs is a more effective bone stimulus than walking? That is because you generate more G-impact and stretch your tendons more with every step down.*

PULL YOUR SOCKS UP *****

BALANCE/ COORDINATION (2 CALS/MIN)

Here's something you didn't know: Astronauts in space put their pants on both legs at a time! How do you put yours on and take them off? And how do you put on and take off your shoes, socks, or pantyhose? Do you lean on something or sit down—or can you do it while standing up without holding onto anything? Do you place your heel on your other knee for balance? What you ultimately want to aim for is to maintain your erect posture and bring the foot up as high as you can. This way you'll be building the best balance skills. My good friend Judy tells me I owe her a lot of money for the pantyhose she tore when she was working on mastering this habit! It is a small price to pay for regaining good balance.

Morning and evening, try to improve your technique when you put on and take off your socks, shoes, and trousers. You will be amazed at your progress within two weeks. This is one of the best and easiest habits you can build into your daily activities to improve your overall balance, and it couldn't be more convenient. You are going to be getting dressed and undressed anyway, so you might as well use the process to your best advantage! This is the essence of developing the good G-habits that will keep you healthy and mobile your entire life.

When you're ready, you can really challenge your balance by repeating this move—carefully!—with your eyes shut. Without visual cues, you have to rely on good posture. Standing correctly will automatically cause your abdominal muscles to contract, which keeps you from toppling over. You will come to realize how much you depend on your eyes for staying upright, instead of using your sense of gravity.

IN THE KITCHEN ****

Preparing a meal from scratch involves standing, reaching, bending, and many motions of the arms and wrists as you wash, slice, chop, stir, lift pots and pans, or roll out cookie dough. Using a manual can opener gives benefits, too. Enjoying foods that must be eaten with a knife and fork, or with chop sticks (as opposed to effort-reducing finger foods like pizza, wraps, and burgers) involves an effort of coordination for the hands and wrists.

USE A BROOM ***

It takes a lot of elbow grease to sweep a floor with a broom. It may be old-fashioned, but it's quiet and thorough. Plus, it's energy efficient, reaches into every corner, and sweeps your stress away. After a light snowfall, I use a broom instead of the shovel. It does a much better job, and it is quiet and fun.

BOOK ON HEAD ****

POSTURE/ BALANCE/ SPINE (1–10 CALS/MIN)

Think of the women in many developing countries who carry jugs of water back from the well on their heads. Don't you envy their erect posture and strong spines? Though most of us do not have to carry water on our head, we can form the same habit. Begin by placing a small bean bag on your head; next, place a small book on your head while sitting in a straight-backed chair. Working at your computer is a good start. If you slouch or raise your shoulders, the book will fall off. Once you've mastered balancing the book while sitting still, carry it on your head as you walk around. You will get better at this with perseverance and the activity's star rating will rise. You may increase the size and weight of the book, making it a spine-strengthening habit as well.

A variation is to make a game of it, especially if you have children or grandchildren in the house. Timing how long one can keep a plastic bowl of water from falling is a great game for young and old. Failure means getting wet! Children may find it harder to do sitting down because they will have to sit still. Now there's a challenge!

HEAD-DOWN POSITION *****

GETS BLOOD TO THE HEAD

Caution: *Do not do this if you have glaucoma or high blood pressure without first checking with your doctor.*

I remember being very upset when my teenage kids would loll in their beloved bean bag chairs, feet up in the air, "doing homework!" They probably did a great deal of good to their brains. It is said that 20 percent of the body's daily energy is used by the brain, and most of it is for basic maintenance of its neurons. The brain does not make its own glucose, so it depends on blood to transport oxygen and glucose to the neurons, the brain's nerve cells you want to keep healthy. The oxygen is needed to burn the glucose and so provide the energy to make the proteins the brain needs to function. Thus, spending limited amounts of time in a head-down position helps the brain remain plastic, forming new cells and connections and staying young.

Another way to get blood to the head is to exercise vigorously enough for the heart to pump more blood up there. Did you ever notice how children seem to spend so much time with their head down, looking through their legs? Try it yourself. Hang head-down on the parallel bars. Sleep with one pillow, or none. Do the next best thing to a shoulder-stand: Lie on your back, legs up, then push your hips up, supported by your hands, upper back, and shoulders. I remember when I was a child my friends and I would hang over the side of the bed or couch to play a board game or read a book. It feels so good. Why did we ever stop doing that?

SWINGS AND ROCKING CHAIRS * TO ****

BALANCE/ FUN (1–4 CALS/MIN)
You are never too old to play, so why not go to the park and swing on a swing? Rediscover the thrill. How high can you go? It is a great acceleration stimulus for your inner ear and balance. Instead of meeting your friends at a restaurant, organize a swing picnic! Or meet your friends at a playground for an hour after school to play and supervise children that may join you. Both children and parents will love you for it and it is a great intergenerational activity. If no one shows up, you get the swings to yourself!

Even just rocking in a rocking chair, though obviously not as powerful, still provides gravity benefits to the mechanism in the inner ear that helps us maintain balance and orient ourselves to our surroundings. I wonder whether this is why babies like being rocked—to stimulate their inner ear?

DANCE

A) JITTERBUG *****
STAMINA/ BALANCE/ LEG MUSCLES/ BLOOD PRESSURE (270–300 CALS/HR)
What more enjoyable way is there to stay fit than dancing? If you haven't danced in years, put on some music in the privacy of your living room and see how you hold up after three or four numbers—especially if it is something energetic like the salsa, jitterbug, or polka. Ballroom dancing may look sedate, but when done with good form it is surprisingly taxing.

B) Folk Dancing *****
Stamina/ Bladder Control (270–300 cals/hr)

A friend told me about a bouncy dance step she learned in a Balkan folk dancing class: With each small, quick step, you allow your upper body to bounce in rhythm. When you have it right, you'll feel the rapid up-down momentum in your chest and upper back. This dance has the added benefit of helping tremendously with another gravity casualty—bladder strength. *SELF* magazine reported in January 2009 about a *JAMA* report that roughly 10 percent of people ages 20 to 39 suffer from incontinence due to pelvic floor disorder, the condition in which pelvic muscles are weakened by weight gain or childbirth. Other folk dance styles, such as Irish step dancing, provide similar benefits.

Play a Musical Instrument or Conducting ** to*****
Stamina/ Upper Body Muscle Strength (240–300 cals/hr—Add 120 more cals burned for standing if conducting = 400 cals/hr)

The rewards depend on which instrument you play and how much energy and practice you put into your playing. Top musicians live to a ripe old age and continue performing—think of Heifetz, Rubinstein, and Rostropovitch. Many switch to conducting as well, which is very physically taxing. You only have to watch Zubin Mehta or Loren Maazel to appreciate the intensity of their concentration and effort. If you cannot play an instrument, how about learning to play one? Or, stand up and conduct the best you can while watching the maestro on TV conducting a famous orchestra.

Play a Sport * to ***
Eye-Hand Coordination/ Muscles/ Bones/ Stamina

Golf, for instance? Excellent! It gets you out socializing and breathing fresh air. Do you carry your own golf clubs from shot to shot? If you do, it's great weight-training (300 cals/hr)! If you are not up to this level of fitness, at least consider forgoing the electric golf cart. Even if you hire a caddy or pull your golf bag on wheels, you'll be getting some excellent walking exercise, along with swinging your clubs.

You can make just about any sport into a habit, and it will provide great practice for your hand-eye coordination and balance. Most sports will

Romancing Your Clubs

At 72, the famous writer John Updike was still working on improving his golf game. Though his wife may have thought he was doing it for macho reasons, he saw the romantic side of carrying his clubs. "I like having the clubs kind of wrapped around me," he said. "I like being close to the clubs, and I like walking up to the ball instead of zigzagging toward it in a cart.... Ideally I like to walk and carry. You want to get some health benefit out of this; otherwise it's all exasperation and disappointment."

stimulate arms, legs, hips, and stamina. To play a sport correctly—golf or tennis, for instance—depends on learning to take advantage of gravity. The correct pendular motion of a golf or tennis stroke depends on letting your arm track gravity. Playing table tennis or snooker also sharpens hand-eye coordination. In climbing or hiking, you propel your weight up a slope, working against the force of gravity.

A sport will also give you aerobic fitness, depending on how much you exert yourself, which translates into stamina and endurance. How hard your heart pumps, how high you send your heart rate, and how long you can keep it up are all measures of how much oxygen you take in—your aerobic effort. You may stroll or you may power walk, you may take a leisurely bike ride or pedal harder, you may swim laps, use a rowing machine or kayak, skip rope, ski, skate, play badminton or volleyball, or dance. If your heart rate increases, that's an aerobic exercise, and if you keep at it, you will build stamina and endurance. Eventually, as you grow fitter, your heart rate will not go up as high when doing the same amount of work and you will be able to sustain your effort longer. This indicates your level of cardiovascular fitness, though not necessarily your strength.

An additional note about swimming is needed. As a competitive swimmer in my youth, I confess to my bias, but swimming is one of the kindest

Tennis for Life

Make sport a habit and you can play for your entire life. Henry Zalzal, a former Egyptian Davis Cup player, enjoyed a good game of singles. At 83, on doctor's orders, he was allowed to play tennis doubles every day before having a light lunch with his partners.

yet most effective exercises you can do. It spares your joints from injury by unweighting your body. Anyone, at any age, and many persons with disabilities, can do it. However, to get the most out of swimming means using it as a sport—swimming laps, resisting the water with each stroke, or walking against the force of the water to tone up muscles and build up aerobic fitness. Unfortunately, there is a mistaken belief that by merely sitting in water we derive some benefit. The reverse is true, since it is much like being in the gravity-free environment of space.

At the end of one of my talks, a 45-year old volunteered that he had once been a skip-rope champion, but he had never thought of taking it

G-BENEFITS OF POPULAR SPORTS	
Sport	**G-Benefit**
Tennis, racquetball, badminton, squash	Balance, coordination, strength, stamina
Table tennis, shooting pool	Hand-eye coordination, stamina
Rowing, kayaking	Stamina, strength, balance
Skateboarding, snowboarding, surfing, skating, skiing	Acceleration, balance and coordination, strength, stamina
Walking, hiking, mountain climbing	Impact loading, acceleration, stamina, strength
Bicycling	Acceleration, balance and coordination, stamina
Hop, skip, playing hopscotch, skip rope, jump, trampoline	Vertical increased gravity load, impact, balance and coordination, stamina
Swimming, diving, fly-fishing	Stamina, coordination, strength—gentle on joints
Tumbling: tripod, tip-up, somersaults, head stand, handstand, cartwheel, parallel bars, slide, see-saw	Balance and coordination, acceleration, inversion gets blood to the head, flexibility. Remember doing these in school? I did not suggest these but you are welcome to try if you have kept up your fitness. Please do not hurt yourself!

> **Tip:** *Make it fun. If you've got a rowing machine, combine your rowing with a favorite travel destination. Get a map and track your progress in rowing miles. You will be in Fiji in no time.*

up again. He left with a determined look to rediscover fun. You may not be able (or want) to play hopscotch any more, but make sure you try at least to stand on one leg. If you can add a little hop, so much the better. If you can negotiate a hop, keep it up, and you may be able to jump soon. Try jumping jacks again if your joints will let you. Start with a few and gradually increase your stamina, smiling and singing all the time. If you play tennis, jumping jacks are a must to get your feet moving—same for that split-step so crucial to good volleying. Learn to ride a bicycle if, like me, you never learned as a child. Tour your neighborhood, or ride back and forth to work every day—you'll be amazed at how much more of the scenery, houses, gardens, gazebos, and mailboxes you can take in from a bike than from whizzing past in a car.

Don't forget to Pray *to ****

Whatever your faith, most religions have a physical expression of prayer. It can range from an upright rocking motion or kneeling once a day to the more elaborate Muslim genuflection five times a day. A recent Malayasian study found significant medical benefits on the cardiovascular system, blood, as well as muscle and bone resulting from the *solat* daily prayer.[4] Five times a day, starting at dawn and ending at sunset, each *solat* consists of 2, 4, 4, 3, and 4 bowing units, or *raka't*, respectively, for a total of 17 per day. This is very close to our findings that it takes at least 16 changes per day from lying down to standing up and back to prevent the space-like physiological changes induced by lying in bed the rest of the time.[5]

Some Everyday G-Habits

Shop in Stores ** (130–160 cals/hr) rather than through the Internet. By moving around instead of sitting in front of the computer, you'll be getting the benefits of walking, reaching for items on shelves, and carrying packages. Your eyes will feast on the visual displays in shop windows. You will see other shoppers, what they look like, what they are wearing or not wearing…and you may even make a new friend or two.

Tip: Develop your own habits list. Rediscover the joy of doing things for yourself as well as for others. The point is not to show off that you can do whatever you used to, but that you can rediscover the joy of playing and being active. How about flying a kite?

Walk in the Mall *** **(150–300 cals/hr)** before it opens. Many people do this now, especially to stay out of the cold in the winter. Some malls even have a "mall-walkers" group. The stores are closed, so it costs you nothing.

Stimulate your Brain *** **(84–110 cals/hr)** by learning something new—a language, bridge or some other game, how to do your taxes on your own—ah, the satisfaction! You'll be stimulating your nerve connections. MRI studies show increases in brain blood flow and metabolism in people doing crossword puzzles, even though the calorie consumption is modest. The hippocampus memory cells light up with energy when one is doing recall exercises.

Do something all day long, every day. Don't believe that because you exercised for 30 minutes or an hour three or five days a week you have fulfilled your daily gravity requirement. If you are watching TV, make a point of doing something during commercial breaks. Do a couple of controlled stand-ups or touch your toes—your brain will thank you—and be sure to sit down slowly to make your leg muscles and bones stronger.

BE A CHILD AGAIN

Oh, yes you can! Bring out the child in you! Rediscover the joy of playing, the feel of your body getting stronger, and your chest swelling with pride and satisfaction at taking that first independent step. Why not? What stops you? Are you afraid to make a fool of yourself? Who cares? Remember learning how to ski? What about riding a bicycle? I had my first go at 60! The neighbors, including a Michigan congressman, turned out to watch this phenomenon. Pretty soon passers-by stopped as well and a laugh was had by one and all as they shouted, "Go! Go!" When I could more or less keep my balance, I tried a right turn. It took a while before I mastered the left turn. What fun! It opened up a whole new experience and it was so good for my balance.

High-frequency, low-intensity, habitual, stop-and-start activities throughout the day are the path to health. They make the most of gravity, and by their very nature include limitless varieties of movements that benefit your whole body. You will slim down, too. Just add up how many calories you would burn with all these activities throughout the day and you will find that they total more than you can burn during your workout. Even when you sit or sleep you can burn up to 60–100 cals/hr. Because of their relatively low intensity and being spread out throughout the day, these movements lend themselves to becoming lifelong habits. They are easy to sustain because they contribute to an effortless way of life.

THE RETURN OF THE CLOTHESPIN

Hanging out clothes to dry can increase flexibility and arm strength as you raise the wet clothes overhead, and then reach and bend down for more. In England, there is a move back to hanging out clothes on a line to dry instead of using the electric dryer. The sale of clothespins, or pegs, soared in the first half of 2007. The Energy Savings Trust and councils across the country are promoting the return of the peg, not for better health and fitness, but on the basis of saving money, and our planet. Using a dryer for every wash is said to be responsible for emitting about 140Kg of CO_2 per year, not to mention the motivation from the $140 saved in the cost of energy. Stretching up to hang out wet clothes and collecting them later all add to the cumulative movement credit. Though discouraged in many U.S. suburban communities, it is certainly practiced in rural areas. Lately, the Sierra Club has organized a "right to dry" movement in many states to encourage hanging clothes out to dry as an energy-saving move.

CHAPTER 4 NOTES

1. Adapted from selected MET values created by B. E. Ainsworth, W. L. Haskell, M. C. Whitt, M. L. Irwin, A. M. Swartz, et al. "Compendium of physical activities: An update of activity codes and MET intensities." *Medicine and Science in Sports and Exercise* 32 (9):S498–504, 2000.

2. Hardy, S. E., Perera, S., Roumani, Y. F., Chandler, J. M., Studenski, S. A. "Improvement in usual gait speed predicts better survival in older adults." *J Amer Geriatrics Soc.* 55(11):1727–1734, 2007.

3. Moffatt, M., Lewis, C. B. *Age-Defying Fitness: Make the Most of Your Body for the Rest of Your Life.* Peachtree Publishers, Georgia, 2006.

4. Abdullah Ahmed Badawi, Prime Minister of Malaysia, in *The New Straits Times*, December 13, 2006.

5. Vernikos, J., Ludwig, D. A., Ertl, A. C., Wade, C. E., Keil, L. C., O'Hara, D. "Effect of standing or walking on physiological changes induced by head down bed rest." *Aviat Space Env Med* 67:1069–1079, 1996.

5

Activity, Exercise, and Gravity Machines

In the search for health and fitness, huge emphasis has been placed on intensive exercise performed in a relatively short period of time and designed primarily to build stamina and, to a lesser extent, strength. But let's face it: Most of us are not training to be elite athletes. Though the numbers of people competing in marathons have increased in recent decades, they are still but a drop in the ocean. Nor can (or should) people keep training at that level for the rest of their lives, not least because of injuries and worsening bone loss. The assumption that this endurance exercise prescription suffices and replaces what our ancestors did throughout the day has been proven incorrect. As Gerry Reaven of Stanford University concluded in 2001, "…. the importance of habitual physical activity, as distinct from exercise training, …should no longer be minimized."[1]

Up to this point I have talked mostly about the benefits of using non-exercise, NEAT-type activities to strengthen your body and increase your metabolism through gravity. But how does that fit in with the many types of exercise vying for our time and attention: aerobic or anaerobic, isotonic, as in weight-lifting, and resistive or isometric, where muscles are put under tension by pushing against each other or onto something fixed? They all seem to be important. If you had to choose one, which would it be? Then there is the issue of duration. It used to be that 30 minutes a day was the ideal, yet we are also told that only 10 minutes might be enough. "Enough" for what? These approaches to fitness all seem important and they work in different ways on different systems.

Yet, if you want to be prepared for the real challenges in life—getting off the couch without help, standing on a ladder to prune a tree, running down the stairs of your hotel when the fire alarm goes off in the middle of the night, lifting your document-filled carry-on into the overhead compartment of your plane, or running across an airport to make your connection—training with exercise machines may not be the way to go. "Consider the physical trainer who employs exercise machines to isolate muscles versus the trainer who prefers to use free weights in training. The first trainer is exercising experimental control, whereas the second is not. The free-weight trainer knows that in everyday life you cannot use isolated muscle groups. When a heavy box you are carrying shifts, you have to compensate for that shift with abs and back muscles and legs," write Landy and Conte in their book *Work in the 21ˢᵗ Century*.[2]

There's nothing wrong with traditional structured exercises, *as long as you use them in addition to your all-day activity G-habits.* If you feel the need to go to the gym, by all means do so, but do so only to supplement your habits. In this way, if for any reason you stop working out, you will always have your G-habits to maintain your basic level of fitness.

The Health and Fitness Pyramid

I like to think of the relationship between non-exercise G-habits on the one hand, and exercise on the other, like a pyramid—or, perhaps more attractively, like an ice cream sundae. Non-exercise G-habits are the ice cream, or the base of the pyramid. You can add toppings as you wish, but without that ice cream underneath, it isn't a sundae. Think of different levels of exercise as chocolate syrup, whipped cream, and a cherry—they are fine on top of your basic G-habits, as long as you don't go overboard with them and maintain the G-habit foundation underneath.

As you saw in Chapter 4, it is all-day non-exercise activity that:

- gives you the most overall health return for your effort

- you are least likely to stop if you cannot remain motivated, are injured, or find yourself strapped for time, energy, or money; and

- is least likely to result in injury or other undesired consequences.

These G-habits are mostly anaerobic, but with a good dose of aerobic activity thrown in, providing the flexibility, strength, balance, coordination, and metabolic energy needed for a healthy body to function within normal limits. This forms the **Basic** (ice cream) level of the pyramid (see the Health and Fitness Pyramid below).

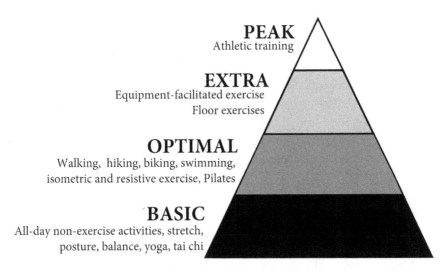

Fig. 2. The Health and Fitness Pyramid

I have included yoga in this foundation level of the pyramid because, although usually thought of as a floor exercise offered in classes, yoga is actually a practice that can be incorporated as a G-habit throughout the day. Originating from an ancient Hindu practice of connecting mind, body, and spirit, yoga is based on a system of stretching, postures, and breathing exercises, many derived from observing children, animals, and nature—our world's gravity experts. Practicing yoga will help you develop good upright posture, which allows the body, planted squarely on the feet, to resist gravity by stacking or aligning the spinal vertebrae on top of each other and supporting the 15-pound head as if it were pulled straight up away from gravity. The feet are important, because so many of us in the developed world spend day after day with our feet forced into uncomfortable shoes.

Yoga is the only exercise discipline that emphasizes getting the blood to the head through a variety of head-down positions. These include simple passive lying on the back, legs supported against a wall, or the advanced head-stand we associate with traditional yoga. There is a reason these are called restorative poses. Whatever our aptitude level, they allow us to relax totally and achieve an incredible sense of calm. Yoga is the discipline that most comprehensively uses gravity to stimulate all parts of the body. It is thermogenic, like the NEAT activities, and generates energy.

77

The more proficient you become at doing the moves correctly, the more benefits you derive. However, there are no good caloric burn estimates. Stretching moves can burn as much as 180 cals/hour. Many yoga moves, like sun salutations, are aerobic stamina-building activities, as evidenced by the increased heart rate; these could burn as much as 300 cals/hr.

Most yoga moves are isometric, or they increase flexibility through holding a gentle stretch. This is key because the *first step* to preventive health care is maintaining or increasing your flexibility. Why is flexibility so important? Because decreased flexibility is the first sign of inactivity or aging. If you no longer can touch your toes with knees straight from a standing position, you've got some work to do. Fortunately, yoga can restore your flexibility painlessly.

Yoga also introduces the concept of using gravity for complete relaxation. Though not considered an exercise, yoga is a fundamental aspect of making all activity efficient and effective. Our natural relaxation—sleep—whether at night or during a nap, was designed to allow our body to totally give in to gravity. This frequently does not actually happen because residual stress and muscle tension can, in fact, carry over into sleep, causing it to be disturbed. Relaxation is now incorporated into all yoga exercise classes, though it is not always explained how it is best achieved. Giving in to gravity with a sense of one's total body weight, head-to-toe, being drawn with abandon to the center of the Earth, is the only way to achieve total, restorative relaxation. We have yoga to thank for that. Relaxation is as essential to good health and optimal performance of muscles and other organs as activity itself.

Balance is another significant part of staying healthy. In the foundation of the pyramid, I also included the ancient art of t'ai chi ch'uan (popularly referred to as tai chi), which is practiced to this day in many lands where the Chinese left their cultural imprint. You will see practitioners gather in the early morning from the garden squares of Hong Kong to the streets of San Francisco. Tai chi is characterized by a series of very slow, flowing, ballet-like, deliberate movements requiring concentration and good balance. It probably works primarily on the body's system of stabilizer muscles, which, as described in chapters 3 and 4, are those that work continuously at a low grade to keep the body upright against gravity and therefore maintain balance. Studies, using a test of balancing on one leg, found that persons aged 60–85 who practiced tai chi did better than those who did not. In particular, they had half the incidence of falls when compared with a group of regular exercisers. Tai chi is now used for restoring balance and in the rehabilitation of stroke patients.

OPTIMAL FITNESS

The second level of the pyramid—the whipped cream on the ice cream—takes you to **Optimal** health and fitness, all within the course of your day. Here I have put aerobic activity like walking, biking, or swimming, all of which give greater stamina. Also, activities like squatting to pick up something, holding the squeeze on a tennis ball, holding a muscle

---

A TECHNIQUE TO ACHIEVE COMPLETE RELAXATION

Here's a description of a method that might help you achieve complete, whole-body gravity relaxation:

Lie on your back with eyes shut. Relax as deeply as you can. Now, starting at your toes and feet, contract them as tightly as you can and then let go; think about gravity pulling them down. Feel the weight of your heels sinking through the floor. Holding onto that feeling, slowly move up to your calves and repeat this sequence, feeling their weight, giving in to gravity pulling and pushing you downward. Move up to your hips and lower back, and feel your abdomen pulled downward. Move further up, feeling the weight of your chest and shoulders sinking into the floor. Feel the knots in your shoulders and neck let go and dissolve. Move up to your head. Let go of all 15 pounds of it. Feel your scalp and your hair slide downward. Scrunch up all your face muscles and let go. Let your jaw drop and your cheeks, tongue, eyes, and forehead slide down. Let all thoughts on that slate be erased by gravity. Everything can wait. Nothing is more important at this moment. Now you are in total relaxation. Relish the moment a good long time. Don't even worry about your breathing. It will happen anyway.

I do not believe I ever achieved complete and total relaxation until by chance I started thinking of gravity pulling me downward as I lay on the floor. Being told to "sink" into the floor or "relax" did not quite do it for me. It turns out that I still had parts of my body like my eyes, jaw, scalp, and skin that only totally let go when I started thinking "gravity." You may say, "What does this have to do with strength and health?" Recovery from exertion against the force of gravity is a very important factor in the effectiveness of the activity.

---

contraction in your thighs or arms during a boring meeting, or sucking in your abdominal muscles at the traffic lights can add lean strength to leg, hand, arm, and stomach muscles. Any activity that lifts up, pushes up, or pulls up your body weight, such as standing up, climbing, hiking, or squatting, increases both stamina and strength.

It is estimated that at least 60 percent of our skeletal muscles are devoted to opposing gravity.[3] The best strength-training exercise relies on your supporting or lifting your own body weight, thus working against the force of gravity. As muscles contract, so do ligaments and tendons that in turn pull on bones, stimulating bone growth. Nerve endings in your feet, legs, buttocks, and spine send signals to tell your brain the whereabouts of your body and its parts and to keep your sense of direction sharp. Depending on your orientation, your blood may shift to your feet, hands or head, exercising heart and blood vessels, gut, and bladder, which are also muscles.

As we mature and age, we lose muscle. Specifically, during every 10 years of adulthood, men lose about seven pounds of muscle and women lose five pounds. Less muscle slows down metabolism. The strength training described above has been shown to reverse much of this muscle loss, and it brings on many benefits—decreased insulin resistance, reduced

THE MUSCLE-BONE PARTNERSHIP

Bones need the loading provided by body weight to become denser, but muscles tell them where the new bone should go. Astronauts returning from months in space on the International Space Station have lost both muscle and bone. Once back on Earth, muscles are rebuilt much faster than bone. This can become a problem because stronger muscles are now pulling on thinner bone and can cause fractures. Astronauts are eager to recover their strong muscles and previous high level of fitness, but rehabilitation doctors have to slow down their enthusiasm in order to allow bones a chance to rebuild normally. If you have not exercised for many years and decide to start up again, you may also be vulnerable to fractures at first, though your exercise will protect your bones in the long run. A Swedish study followed 2,205 men for 35 years, beginning at age 49–51. About one quarter of the men eventually suffered hip fractures. Not too surprisingly, the men who maintained the highest level of overall activity had the fewest fractures.

arthritic pain, lower resting blood pressure, and more. It even improves memory by increasing brain blood flow (though not as easily as exercises with your head in a downward position). Weight-training does not work without gravity, so weight is crucial to its effectiveness. Strength training can be as good as weight training, but it works by using resistance, instead. Since astronauts are essentially weightless in space, their exercise devices use resistance (strength) training. However, even resistance training does not wholly protect astronauts in space nor, in fact, volunteers lying in bed continuously. There is more to gravity than merely providing weight.

Another form of strength training came from what is now known after its inventor. Joseph Pilates (1880–1967), a German citizen interned in England during World War I, applied his own version of yoga techniques to wounded soldiers lying in bed. The purpose was to teach them to exercise their trunk muscles in order to remain in good shape. Many of these men could not stand up to use their body weight, nor were they able to lift weights, but they could contract their trunk muscles. This conditioning regimen, although it bypassed working against gravity, also helped them improve their posture and muscle strength when they got out of bed.

Strong abdominal muscles are crucial for a healthy back. The large lower abdominal muscle, the *transverse abdominus*, that runs across the base of the abdomen and wraps all the way around to the back, supports the spine, but it is a muscle that is hard to tone. When it sags as fat accumulates in the abdomen, it pulls your spine forward or sideways, a major cause of back pain. This lower abdominal is the muscle that contracts when you give a hearty belly laugh, are mildly constipated, sneeze, exhale hard, and grunt excessively, like tennis champion Maria Sharapova. It can also make or break your sexual pleasure. The best exercise to tone this muscle depends on learning to *engage* and keep the abdominal muscles contracted as much as you can throughout the day to strengthen them and help you maintain good posture.

Muscles that support the shoulder blades and upper spine become overstretched by slouching. They can be contracted and toned in the same

> *Tip:* For strength training place greater emphasis on correct form, tightening all muscles, holding longer, and allowing for recovery. Keep breathing!

way. Couple these contractions with a forced Pilates exhalation—one loud enough to hear—emptying your lungs as much as possible, and you will be working these elusive abdominal muscles as well. I do mine while waiting at traffic lights!

Holding tension and contraction can also be achieved with isometric activities that strengthen muscles by using tension bands, pushing or pulling hands against each other or against a stationary object. Your muscles contract when you lift a weight, but you may also contract them by simply imagining you are lifting a weight or by pushing against some solid object while holding still.

The mind is a powerful tool. You can actually strengthen muscles by willing and visualizing your muscles to contract. You can also achieve a result similar to that of lifting weights by voluntarily contracting those muscles that would have had to contract if you were actually lifting that weight. The advantage of these exercises is that you can do them anywhere, anytime. The benefit depends on how hard you try and how long you hold the contraction. You will find that exhaling as you contract helps a lot. One such useful exercise is called the Kegel. This is one of the safest, most effective treatments for urinary incontinence (UI). Though known for a long time to help women with UI, after prostate surgery, men may find it helpful as well. Identify your pelvic muscles when you urinate by contracting around your rectal area to interrupt your urine flow. Then any time you think of it during the day or on that long airplane ride, squeeze those muscles tight for 5–10 seconds without holding your breath and then slowly relax. You can also do short, repetitive squeezes that last only two seconds. They are good for your sex life as well.

Isometric exercise is excellent when you do not have the time, space, or equipment to do weight training, and you may do them either standing up or sitting down. For instance, while stopped at traffic lights is a great time to contract abdominal muscles, while exhaling hard and slowly. (Note that this is not such a good idea while you are driving.) These exercises are also great for long airplane travel or while watching TV.

The idea is that you contract hard, hold as long as you can, and relax completely. As with the weight-training exercises, allowing time for recovery is very important with isometrics.

You can also get a great deal of benefit through tensing up parts or all of your body and holding the tension. If you ever feel cold, contracting your muscles in this way warms you up in a flash. That is why these actions are called thermogenic—they generate heat. They are very energizing and can be done anywhere, with no equipment. Feeling sleepy during a meeting or a talk? Energize!

As you can see, there are a wide variety of options you can choose from to strengthen your muscles and energize yourself throughout the day, literally anywhere, with no facilities or equipment required.

The Optimal level of the Health and Fitness Pyramid provides the level of health and fitness that allows you to enjoy participating throughout your life in your favorite sport as an adult or to be sought out by your classmates and enjoy team sports as a child. But, most of all, this level of fitness is all you need to stay in top health even if you slip up at times.

EXTRA

Anything above optimal is **Extra**, the chocolate sauce drizzled on top of the whipped cream. Designed to build up muscle mass by pumping iron, increase stamina even further as a foundation to a higher level of sport activity, or achieve some cosmetic benefit, these exercises include outdoor jogging—which is not too kind on your joints—or require equipment mostly found in a gym or intense floor exercise classes. Unsupervised, these are most likely to result in injury. Endurance activities, in particular, if overdone with zeal, may backfire even in young, fit, and healthy persons.

Structured fitness programs such as those in a gym are based mainly on aerobics and strength training, with a little balance and flexibility training thrown in. They rely on different types of exercise and the use of machines to benefit your body in different ways. For even greater effectiveness, you must always increase their intensity. The primary advantage of going to the gym is that its very structured approach helps maintain motivation, especially for those who can afford a personal trainer.

However, there are downsides. A typical gym program will miss out on working most muscles in your body. Then, too, many people find it hard to set aside the time, and may consider it expensive or embarrassing. And the benefits are lost very rapidly once you stop.

You may also choose to exercise in the privacy of your home. There are plenty of floor exercise videos, books, magazines like *SELF*, and Internet programs that promise lithe, leaner bodies, as long as you persevere.

However, much like dieting, few do persevere. As with the daily non-exercise activities listed in Chapter 4, addressing these "extra" exercises from a gravity perspective should help you sort out which ones are best for you.

Handheld free weights are the most commonly used form of weight training. In contrast to whole-body weight activities, these weight exercises benefit only specific muscles. Get smart about your workouts. Some exercise combinations include more than one move to target multiple muscles, and may feature moves above your head to make them more gravity-efficient. It is highly advisable to begin by doing these exercises only with appropriate supervision, because you may injure yourself if you do exercises with handheld weights incorrectly. It is very important that you keep your body in an evenly balanced stance. Remember to allow time for recovery after these exercises.

The Danger of Overdoing a Good Thing

My son's friend Wayne is a very healthy 42-year old who enjoys cycling and mountain biking in the mountains of Colorado. Recently, wearing all his protective gear, he was enjoying a beautiful spring day with a bike ride on a familiar country road. Seemingly out of nowhere he was hit from behind by a car.

Wayne was severely injured and rushed to the nearest hospital, where scans and subsequent surgery showed unexpected advanced osteoporosis of the vertebrae. Doctors told him he was a lucky man for two reasons. First, his vertebrae crumbled on impact instead of severing or damaging the spinal cord. The injury that was fully expected to leave him a paraplegic was avoided. A synthetic protective sleeve placed around the spinal cord did the rest. Second, Wayne now knows he has osteoporosis, a condition that would most likely not have been diagnosed until he was older and it became much more severe. Wayne is gradually returning to his usual, active life.

Although osteoporosis has long been recognized in young female distance runners, it has been attributed to eating and menstrual disorders.[4] Much to my surprise, I later learned that osteoporosis of the spine is increasingly observed in young male athletes as well. The causes are still being investigated, one promising theory being the loss of calcium in perspiration.[5]

Handheld weights are those dumbbells you can buy at any sporting goods store for $20 or less. The amount of weight you use should be less than maximal, but heavy enough to engage your muscles, maybe 3–8 pounds. Begin by trying the exercises with various weights until you find the weight that challenges you but does not force you into a bad posture, such as raising your shoulders or stooping forward.

There is an incredible array of machines now available to target various muscles. As with weights, supervision and performing the exercises correctly are extremely important to prevent injury, especially if you are just starting out with this sort of workout. The problem is that individuals tend to follow the same sort of routine over and over again, targeting the same muscles at the exclusion of others.

PEAK

Finally, for the very small segment of those that are (or aspire to be) marathon runners or elite athletes, there exists high level, structured training designed to achieve **Peak** performance—the cherry on top of the sundae.

Note: While people in the Extra or Peak levels of the Health and Fitness Pyramid are in top shape, if for some reason they stop training, their fitness will take a nosedive—unless they also have developed a foundation of basic and optimal activities to fall back on. They cannot afford to slip up.

FUEL FOR YOUR BODY

Is the ice cream sundae analogy making you hungry? Regardless of which level of the Activity Pyramid is right for you, you need to eat. It turns out that there are certain eating habits that, like G-habits, can give you extra benefits.

For that extra muscle-building benefit, *when* you fuel up makes a difference. Your body is an energy-producing/energy-consuming machine. It stands to reason that you need some ready fuel for exercise to protect your body from breaking down muscle. Eat something before you start your most intense habit such as mowing, gardening, or playing tennis; or before you exercise, whatever time of day that might be. This also gives a greater boost to your metabolism.

Several studies have now shown that *eating soon after exercising* is even more important in preventing the counterproductive effect of breaking down muscle tissue. This is especially true after weight training, when both muscle breakdown and rebuilding are going on at a higher rate. A Finnish study found that this rebuilding process increases by 21 percent up to three hours after weight training exercise, whereas muscle breakdown increases by 17 percent. These data agree with Peter Raven's work, which indicates that metabolism stays elevated for up to four hours after weight training.[6] Longer after-effects have been reported, though absolute conclusions are questionable since the conditions of each study—such as the type, intensity, and duration of exercise, and the gender and age of trained or untrained subjects—tend to vary greatly with each study. However, it seems generally agreed that consuming protein or amino-acids, particularly what are called branched-chain amino acids like leucine, during or soon after exercise, stimulates muscle protein synthesis after both resistance-type or aerobic exercise.[7]

Ideally, you should eat something within 30 minutes of exercising; certainly don't delay longer than two hours. Since you are eating to rebuild muscle—protein synthesis—*what you eat should be rich in amino acids and protein.* Dr. Bill Evans at the University of Arkansas recommends whey, a protein-rich drink that is a by-product of cheese production.[8] It is refreshing and tastes good, and provides an easy, quick source of what you need to rebuild muscle. If drinking whey (or a shake made with whey powder) doesn't appeal to you, you may be glad to know that whey is a main ingredient in yogurt.

GRAVITY MACHINES: PULLING GS

Apart from using your body's own weight to increase gravity stimulus when walking, running and jumping, or by holding weights, there are mechanical devices, known as gravity machines, that you can use to get the same benefits. These devices do not just simply increase the load on the body. They help improve balance, coordination, and blood pressure regulation. Studies of bed-bound volunteers to evaluate these devices' usefulness as therapeutic measures for astronauts have also shown positive effects on muscle function and bone density.[9] Through acceleration, they provide greater directional stimulus to the inner ear and brain centers that process gravity.

By now, I think I've made it clear that there are many different ways one can increase or decrease the gravity load and acceleration stimulus on the whole body and on different parts of the body. *Gravity* is fast becoming a recognized buzzword in the fitness arena, and as a result, equipment and activities have come on the market, claiming their effectiveness through the benefits of gravity. Whether or not they are actually effective depends on what they are compared with. For instance, if you compare an upright exercise with one done lying down, whether it uses a machine or not, the upright vertical gives you maximum G-benefit for muscle, bone, and cardiovascular results. You may enhance the benefit on bone, and probably muscle and circulation, if you apply some vibration to the soles of the feet as well. Sitting or lying flat or on a board at a slant, head-downward, in fact, *reduces* the influence of the G-stimulus relative to the vertical.

THE STABILIZER STATIONARY BICYCLE

There are no machines that target stabilizer muscles specifically. Scientists at Northumbria University in England, Dr. Dorothee Debuse and Professor George Korfmacher, are testing a most intriguing device that they developed, a device that allows the specific recruiting and training of trunk and lumbar-pelvic stabilizers, in particular. It provides a completely new exercise experience, and it works by facilitating exercise:

- at the equivalent of less than 30 percent maximum voluntary contraction
- over prolonged periods of time
- at low frequencies (0.5 to 3 Hz)
- without working against resistance
- using the body's own energy potential and no external energy.

A computer attached to the device calculates optimum parameters, assesses stabilizer performance, and provides auditory or visual feedback to the operator. Tests have confirmed that the movement provided by this device does indeed recruit stabilizers. Since these are the first muscles to atrophy with inactivity, age, or in people with movement disorders, this approach could make a significant contribution to basic health.

HYPERGRAVITY

Enhancement of the gravity cues and the pull of gravity on the body on Earth, known as hypergravity, depends on the principle that the faster any mass moves—*acceleration*—the heavier it becomes. Jump up and down on a scale and the needle will swing wildly, reaching far beyond the line that indicates your normal weight. Go on a whirling ride at an amusement park and you will find yourself pinned to the back of the seat. You will not fall, even if the floor is temporarily removed. That's acceleration and hypergravity. A small amount of acceleration can be achieved by walking, a little more by running or swinging on a swing, and even more by jumping. Riding a bicycle, a motorcycle, or a horse, speeding in a fast car or a sailboat, flying in a small airplane pulling Gs, whizzing downhill on skis or a sled, whitewater rafting, or spinning on a centrifuge all provide stimulation that is greater than 1G—*hypergravity*—and increase the health benefits of gravity exposure, particularly when provided in an alternating mode as these common activities would.

For the Fun of It

We associate most of these G-stimulating activities with fun. I don't know what the scientific explanation is, but there is no doubt that when we seek fun, we spontaneously turn to a gravity kick (yes, even sex). An adrenaline surge, an endorphin high, a host of other hormones, deeper breathing, faster pounding heart, all these and more come pouring out, followed by a wonderful sense of relaxation.

Let's evaluate the benefits of some gravity machines.

Roller Coaster ****

These thrill rides are excellent gravity machines. They provide intermittent higher and lower gravity exposures to acceleration as you roll down and deceleration as you climb up. And what fun it is! Everyone squeals with delight!

Gravity-Healthy Bones

Fighter pilots performing aerial combat maneuvers experience high stress loads on their vertebrae. As the head-to-toe G-force increases, so does the loading on the spine and pelvis. Fiona Naumann at the Edith Cowan University, in Perth, Australia, and her colleagues monitored the bone response of a group of young Royal Australian Air Force fighter pilots on a 12-month, high-performance flight-training course. The G-forces generated were around three to four times Earth's G and resulted in an 11 percent increase in bone density in the upper spine and a 5 percent increase in the pelvis.

GRAVITY IS CHILD'S PLAY

I have long advocated playgrounds for seniors, like those catching on in Finland and Germany. A study from the University of Lapland designed to make activity more fun for young and old encouraged 40 persons between the ages of 65 and 81 to use a specially designed playground. After three months using climbing frames, swings, and seesaws, the participants built muscle, lost fat, and showed improved balance, coordination, and speed of motion.

TRAMPOLINE ****

Did you know that a Finnish study showed that as you bounce on a trampoline you can generate up to 4.5G at your feet? That compares with 1.3G walking, 1.5–2.1G running, and up to 6G for a full jump impact. You probably never thought of a trampoline as a gravity machine, but it is a most effective one.[10] Traditionally enjoyed by children, trampolines are available with safety rails for adults and seniors, as well as for home gyms. They provide excellent exercise and are great for balance, too. Any vertical acceleration also improves bladder control. Skipping rope, playing hopscotch, or dancing the polka are also of great benefit.

HORSEBACK RIDING ****

Horseback riding is fantastic for your posture and balance. Those who have learned how to ride know how fit they must be to do so and how, in turn, riding keeps them in shape and alert. You slouch on a horse at your peril. The mere act of being at one with a moving horse and maintaining balance helps to tone, stretch, and strengthen the rider's back, abdominal, and leg muscles, the very muscles used for walking. And, oh, what joy it is to gallop through the countryside, breathing in the fresh air!

RIDING MACHINES ***

Machines that claim to mimic horseback riding have been designed. These range from a child's rocking horse to those that shake and toss you about to give the feel of riding a bucking horse. Remember those machines outside supermarkets for children who graduated from a rocking horse to riding in a saddle for ten cents?

The Japanese word for horseback riding is *joba*, and that is what the Japanese have called a saddle-like device that is fast becoming one of the hottest fitness trends. Not unlike the children's saddle ride, this adult version is attractive because it does not require much effort. Although the *joba* session of 30 minutes only burns about 100 calories, using it for 15 to 30 minutes a day, three days a week, improves posture, increases metabolism, and tones muscles, according to Matsushita Electric Industrial Co., the Japanese manufacturer. Other manufacturers, like Panasonic, have developed similar machines.

As on horseback, *joba* riders must tighten their abdomens to maintain balance and squeeze their thighs to prevent themselves from falling off the saddle. But it is the forward-back motion and its rhythm and frequency that stimulate the gravity center control and yield the highest benefit.

BALANCE PLATES AND DISCS ***

As I described in Chapter 2, the "gravity receptors" in the soles of your feet and your seat, the stretch receptors called proprioceptors, play a key role in sensing position and responding to gravity. Stimulating these receptors is beneficial in sharpening balance.

Twelve- to 15-inch air-filled discs with smooth tactile bumps on either side are great for improving balance. Standing on the air-filled disc challenges balance and is a bit like standing on a water-bed. The bumps stimulate the soles of the feet as well. Try to stand on such a disc. Support yourself lightly at first, using a chair back until you can balance yourself for as long as possible. You can challenge yourself further by holding your balance while lifting one leg at a time. You get a bonus from the stimulating massage of the soles of your feet through the protrusions on the disc.

I use my disc to sit on, especially when I am working at the computer. The mild instability it generates encourages good posture without being distracting. It is also relaxing to sit on during long drives. It forces balanced sitting, preventing fatigue or back problems.

EXERCISE SHOES ***

More practical for building balance and improving posture are a variety of specially designed shoes, such as Masai Barefoot Technology (MBT), FitFlops, and Skechers Shape-Ups. The manufacturers encourage wearers to work up their usage of these products gradually, and eventually you can wear them all day long, indoors and out. Designed to mimic the way the human foot moves when walking on soft, uneven ground, they massage the foot, while special inserts in the sole of the shoe generate mild instability that forces continuous and spontaneous balance adjustments. This makes the muscles, joints, and bones work, too. Improved posture can be noticed immediately.

HEALTHY FEET—HEALTHY BALANCE

Don Doerr, a brilliant and critical engineer at the Kennedy Space Center, NASA's launch site, was focusing on my shoes as we walked down the street in New Orleans. A lifelong jogger, he recently tore his tendon and was trying to adapt to a run-free life. I explained my happy outcome with my MBTs, but never gave it a second thought until I received this e-mail: "Just a little status update. My bride has been observing my bouncing walk with the MBTs and has decided that it would be good for her. So she bought a pair and was so happy with them she bought another pair. Now she is talking my youngest daughter into these and because she is a poor, starving vet student, I might get to buy those too. Ain't capitalism great?"

MBT shoes were recommended to me after a most painful tendonitis in the arch of my foot kept me off sports for almost a year. Orthotic inserts in my tennis shoes had been of only limited help. I was told by the orthopedic surgeon that I would have to live with this painful handicap for the rest of my life. Now I have proven him wrong. I wear my MBTs without orthotics and I am back on the courts. What is more, my posture has dramatically improved. They must be working by targeting stabilizer muscles.

TAKE A RIDE ON A MOTORBIKE ***

Riding a motorbike, even as a passenger, requires a good sense of balance. In Bermuda, where you cannot rent a car, the only way to get around the island is by renting a motorbike. My husband was brave enough to take on the task, and I clutched onto him for dear life since it was my first attempt. At the end of the day, we were glad to be in one piece, but we felt invigorated. The next day, my stomach muscles were pleasantly sore. The acceleration provided added Gs, stimulated balance, and contracted muscles to maintain balance.

TAKE A RIDE ON A GYROSCOPE ****

If you are anywhere near the Cosmodrome in Manhattan, Kansas, you can have the ride of your life on a gyroscope. Anyone can ride it, but it is a particularly big hit with the study groups of seniors that have been coming through their classes for the past 10 years. I believe there is one at the Space Center in Houston, Texas, as there are at other space museums around the world. For those of you who think of a gyroscope as an instrument used in navigation, a compass or a device to help stabilize the rocking of ships, aircraft, torpedoes, or spacecraft, you are right. Its symmetrical, wheel-like construction, mass, and rapid rotation conserve angular momentum so that its axis of rotation tends to stay pointing in the same direction. This concept was adapted so that the center—roughly the waist—of the human riding it remains fixed relative to gravity. No motor is involved. All movement of the symmetrical, three-ring gimbaled device is powered by the rider, who controls pace and movement by slight shifts in body weight. The rotor simultaneously spins about its axis and can oscillate about the other two axes. This harmonic design moves the body in three-dimensional space, alternating effort and relaxation. The rider thus gets an intermittent whole-body isometric exercise as the body's position relative to the pull of gravity—head-up, down, or at any angle—is constantly changing. No two rides are alike, providing infinite variety involving all parts of the body. Once you master the concept, this is an outstanding all-around gravity machine.

Human gyroscopes such as the Gyrogym are now available on the market for personal use. They are also used in training football players or athletes in other sports who need to maintain their center of gravity at all times as they tackle, while moving sideways or back and forth. In doing this, it seems that this device may work by training primarily the stabilizer muscles. But just as with a trampoline, if you buy one, do make sure it has the required safety features.

Take a Ride On a Centrifuge *****

A centrifuge is the ultimate gravity machine. It is a rapidly rotating device that, by virtue of its centrifugal force, simulates the effects of gravity and acceleration on whoever is riding on it. I think of a spin on a centrifuge as *whole-body weight training*. One day very soon it will be commonplace to see centrifuges at your local gym to make you fit, trim, and strong.

Consensus has not been achieved on the exact duration, frequency, and intensity of daily G-requirements in these environments, but research is continuing. The answer is not far away. It is apparent that, not unlike exercise, an alternating higher and lower G, rather than a sustained gravity stimulus mode, may be most effective. Dr. Charles Knapp at the University of Kentucky and his team of researchers are finding that, just as with exercise, it takes probably less than 30 minutes to achieve good results by lying on a rotating plate, if the dose of gravity, provided by the number of revolutions per minute, is intermittent. The schedule they settled on for improving blood pressure regulation alternates between 2G for 90 seconds and 1.2G for 40 seconds, for a total of 28 minutes, including a warm-up and cool-down period. I am convinced effective results can be achieved in even shorter times. The dose of gravity and accompanying regimen required for muscle toning or for building bone strength may differ. Centrifugation without exercise probably targets stabilizer muscles that have to work harder to maintain posture against gravity.

You could also combine high-intensity exercise, such as rowing, with the higher G-level to build your stamina at the same time. Imagine being able to train both your stabilizer and your mobilizer muscle systems with a centrifuge. Imagine being able to get your daily dose of gravity with such short exposures! I believe that daily exposure to higher G on a centrifuge—hypergravity—with and without exercise will produce equivalent benefits to your usual exercise routine in 1G, *but in a much shorter time*. I have designed just such a centrifuge, primarily for keeping astronauts healthy on their way to Mars and back, or for space tourists like you who may want to go to the moon for their adventure vacation or their honeymoon.

Back on Earth, I hope that one day soon a basic version of my centrifuge design will be built. Until the day when my gravity machines are available in your local gym, or perhaps even in your home, your best strategy is perpetual motion—acquire and practice those good G-habits as part of your daily routine. That way, you will be in top condition to take advantage of a centrifuge or other machine that may someday cut down your exercise time requirement for fitness, muscle, and bone strength, as well as kick-starting your metabolism, all while comfortably lying on a spinning wheel.

CHAPTER 5 NOTES

1. Reaven, G. M. *Insulin Resistance, Compensatory Hyperinsulinemia, and Coronary Heart Disease: Syndrome X Revisited.* In: Jefferson LS, Cherrington AD (eds.,) *Handbook of Physiology.* Section 7: the endocrine systems. Vol II: the endocrine pancreas and regulation of metabolism. New York: Oxford University Press, pp.1169–1197, 2001.

2. Landy & Conte. *Work in the 21st Century: An Introduction to Industrial-Organizational Psychology,* 2nd ed. Wiley-Blackwell, 2007.

3. Clement, G., Gurfinkel, V. S., Lestienne, F., Lipshits, M. I., Popov, K. E. "Changes in posture during transient perturbations in microgravity." *Aviat Space Env Med* 56:666–671, 1985.

4. Karen Birch. Female athlete triad, *BMJ* 330:244–246, 2005.

5. Klesges, R. C., Ward, K. D., Shelton, M. L., Applegate, W. B., Cantler, E. D., Palmieri, G. M., Harmon, K., Davis, J. "Changes in bone mineral content in male athletes. Mechanisms of action and intervention effects." *J AMA*.276(3):226-30,1996; "The Why Files: Scent of an Athlete," accessed 6/10/09 at http://whyfiles.org/055oddball/sweat.html .

6. Peter Raven, personal communication, 2008.

7. Anthony, T. G., McDaniel, B. J., Knoll, P., Bunpo, P., Paul, G. L., McNurlan, M. A. "Feeding meals containing soy or whey protein after exercise stimulates protein synthesis and translation initiation in the skeletal muscle of male rats." *JNutr*, 137(2):357–362, 2007.

8. Evans, W. J., Couzens, G. S. *AstroFit.* New York: The Free Press, 2002.

9. Pavy LeTraon, A., Heer, Narici, M. V., Rittweger, J., Vernikos, J. "From space to earth: advances in human physiology from 20 years of bed rest studies (1986–2006)." *Eur J Appl Physiol* 101:143–194, 2007.

10. http://ezinearticles.com/?Health-Benefits-Of-A-Mini-Trampoline&id=753837 and http://www.needakrebounders.com/CarolsHealth_Bounce.htm.

6

G-Therapy: Help for Specific Problems

The previous chapters of this book have discussed how gravity therapy can improve the health and well-being of people suffering from Gravity Deprivation Syndrome as a result of a sedentary lifestyle. But what if your situation is worse? What if you find it difficult to get out of bed or out of a chair without help? What if you suffer from a debilitating chronic condition or injury that impairs your mobility and saps your strength?

If this is the case, you are likely to be even more gravity deprived than the merely sedentary. My years of research and my background as a physiologist have led me to conclude that many of today's chronic health problems—such as Syndrome-X, diabetes, balance problems, and obesity—can be linked to gravity deprivation. The good news is that these conditions can often be significantly alleviated with a minimum daily dose of G-therapy.

In the first part of this chapter, we will explore various specific problems that would lend themselves to G-therapy. Then we will take a look at how to apply treatment to alleviate these problems through hypergravity and by stimulating gravity receptors.

GRAVITY THERAPY

You are by now well aware of the benefits of using invigorating gravity to improve the health and strength of an otherwise able body. Using gravity to repair health *problems* is merely an extension of the same lessons learned from space, where super-fit astronauts become less healthy by living without gravity.

Our brain-body motor control system depends on gravity to properly function. Using gravity efficiently can promote repair in people whose controls and relay connections have been compromised through injury or disease, or in people who are bed-ridden for an extended period while recovering from a serious illness.

Before I discuss specific conditions, let me first mention the seven essential tenets for optimizing your body's health and quality of life:

1. The state of the body reflects the state of the brain and mind.

2. The brain is plastic. It can find new ways around a problem. It can replace damaged nerve cells (neurons) or generate new neurons in a brain area at any age in response to appropriate stimulation from the rest of the body or stimuli from the surrounding environment.

3. The brain can recruit a neighboring brain area to take on the function of a damaged one. If one sense is damaged, another can take over for it.

4. If the lower body has been injured or lost communication with the brain, the spinal cord is also plastic; it can be repaired or may be programmed to assume some motor function so that the individual may become somewhat mobile, even if coordination is less than perfect.[1]

5. If you have suffered a severe trauma or illness, your chances of eventual full or partial recovery can be greatly improved by doing everything you can to maintain the health of your brain and body, irrespective of your debility. Using gravity can help! As explained in Chapter 3, gravity acts as a direct mechanical stimulus on every cell in the body. It is converted or transduced to a chemical or physical signal to grow, communicate, heal, or divide, and is a powerful ally in the fight against atrophy and degeneration.

6. The sensitivity of receptors and sensors that receive and process gravity information changes if they are gravity-deprived or exposed to hypergravity. This change in gravity threshold must be taken into account in developing an effective gravity prescription.

7. The longer the time period between injury and the initiation of G-therapy, the lower the chances of recovery, and the more time it will take.

Rehabilitation

G-therapy has much to offer in the realm of rehabilitation. The negative physiological changes that occur in astronauts living in the near-zero G of space closely resemble those typically seen in post-surgery patient populations, or in those who have become deconditioned by lengthy illness, bed-ridden geriatric or spinal cord injured patients, or those in casts for bone fractures or muscle or joint injuries.

Though rehabilitation practices today are, in fact, based on restoring gravitational stimulation—such as getting patients out of bed, upright, and walking as early as possible—they have mostly been triggered by economic motives. Recognition of the role of gravity in providing loading and directional cues has been slow in coming. Therefore, many approaches have been only partially based on the detailed understanding of physiology acquired from space research, and their effectiveness has been less than systematic.

From what you have so far read about Gravity Deprivation Syndrome, you can see that being immobilized after an injury also affects the functioning of brain control centers and circuits, and that even after a wound has completely healed, the brain needs more time to recuperate in order to catch up to its pre-injury state. Similarly, when brain connections are interrupted, such as with brain or spinal injury, stroke, or by injury or infection during childhood, the rest of the body rapidly loses its fitness.

Sitting or Intense Exercise Can Shorten Your Life

Telomeres, those little caps at the end of chromosomes that protect your DNA and allow healthy cell division, become shorter with age. They have therefore become a useful indicator of your state of health. Short telomeres have been linked to illness, such as cancer, cardiovascular disease, depression, shorter lifespan, and early death.

The bad news is that research is now showing that people with a sedentary lifestyle also have shorter telomeres. As you might have guessed, physical activity helps you keep those telomeres longer, but only if it is moderate. More exercise is not better. People with high levels of physical activity had, in fact, shorter telomeres, just like those who sat too much. The message is clear: Be active, but don't overdo it if you want to see those grandkids grow up.

Blood pressure regulation, muscles, bones, and nerve-dependent skills are the first to suffer. So often, because primary attention is focused on the injury, peripheral rehabilitation is not started until after the body has been allowed to decondition, making recovery that much slower and more difficult. We know from space and bed-rest studies that such deconditioning is well under way within 24 hours.

Rehabilitation techniques stand to benefit from being informed by the full range of G-therapy possibilities, starting with preventing the onset of deconditioning in the first place, to standing, moving about, and to using specific means of increasing the patient's gravity load, as well as improving his or her sensitivity to gravity.

METABOLIC DISORDERS

Increasing gravity stimulus is anabolic—it stimulates metabolism. Therefore, G-therapy of various types has been shown useful or promising in conditions that result from metabolic disorders. These include obesity and diabetes; muscle wasting, especially resulting from infection such as HIV, and particularly in patients who may be unable to exercise; and osteoporosis, the loss of bone density and reduced bone formation.

HELPING THE BRAIN HELP ITSELF

There are babies who, because of disease or brain injury, are unable to sense gravity or move during the early critical periods of development. The neural networks involved with balance and coordination may not be laid down in the brain, or may be laid down erratically and be improperly programmed. And an adult brain suffering a serious injury is just as vulnerable when the brain centers and programs laid down during development are interrupted. The tragic outcome is evidenced by a lack of coordination, the inability to stand and carry the body's load, problems in muscle and bone development, and other gravity deprivation symptoms.

LIMITING BIRTH BRAIN INJURY

I have often wondered why, despite all our modern medical advances, there still seems to be such a high incidence of otherwise healthy babies suffering brain damage at birth. A detailed review by Drs. Eileen Simon and George Morley published in *Medical Veritas* in 2005 set me thinking. They made a convincing, thoroughly documented argument of the relationship between immediate cord clamping at birth and neonatal brain damage. Their argument is based on the fact that most infants start breathing within seconds of birth. In others, however, this premature clamping interrupts the normal physiological role of the placenta and umbilical cord, which is to perfuse the infant's lungs with oxygenated placental blood until its own lung circulation and breathing are established.

Circulation and an adequate blood volume are essential for respiration. Immediate clamping almost always reduces the infant's blood volume. The authors cite evidence that even apparently normal newborns may be compromised permanently by the low blood volume, low blood pressure, and the hypoxia that follows.

A newborn infant is, in fact, like a returning astronaut who experiences lower blood volume and low blood pressure on standing. However, the astronaut has at least had the opportunity before going into space to develop blood pressure reflexes in Earth's gravity, which, even though compromised by space, signal the heart to pump more blood up to the head.

The infant makes its entrance into a world of gravity from the weightlessness of the womb. It has not yet had the chance to develop blood pressure regulating reflexes. Its heart pumps, but cannot increase its pumping in response to a change in posture because it has never experienced this before. If held upright, gravity would drain the infant's blood toward its feet. That is why extreme care is taken by nurses in the delivery room to maintain the baby in a horizontal position. If, for any reason, the infant's blood volume is reduced and its blood pressure drops, raising its head up could be disastrous.

In 1996, we flew two monkeys for 12 days on a Russian spacecraft. The purpose was to study in greater detail than is possible in astronauts changes in muscles, joints, and bone. On landing in Siberia, the monkeys, who looked lively and healthy, were whisked to Moscow for evaluation by a team of doctors. The first animal was anesthetized for a whole body scan to assess its muscle and bone status. As the doctors picked him up to turn him over, he unfortunately stopped breathing. In vain, they tried to resuscitate him, but could not. The team then noticed that the second flight monkey, seated in his chair awaiting his turn, was showing signs of distress. They at once laid him down. The animal quickly recovered and the team was able to proceed with the rest of the testing as scheduled.

An independent investigation into the cause of the first animal's death concluded that the animal's reflexes were compromised by being in space, as well as by the anesthesia. Although doing fine while it was horizontal, the monkey was unable to respond with an appropriate increase in blood pressure and brain blood flow as it experienced the pull of gravity when it was tilted up and moved. Devastating as the loss of the animal was, it triggered new awareness among the whole medical team of the importance of maintaining astronauts in a horizontal position if emergency care were ever needed immediately after landing.

An infant exposed to gravity for the first time, after immediate cord clamping when blood volume, pressure, brain blood flow, and oxygen are already low, will be extremely vulnerable to inadvertent posture change. Extreme caution in maintaining the infant in a horizontal position must be taken until its body gradually develops the reflex mechanisms it will need to live in gravity.

Developmental Injury

The Petö Institute, a wonderfully creative center in Budapest, Hungary, has for years been training children with cerebral palsy to learn to walk. They use a program of repetitive motor activities that emphasizes strength and flexibility, eight hours a day, five days a week, first in the horizontal position and as soon as possible in the upright position. The children wear a safety harness at first, until they are able to stand on their own. The earlier such exposure to gravity can start, the better the outcome. All of the children benefit, but the results are best for those who start the program before they are three years old. The story of an eight-year-old boy with cerebral palsy, Blaine Mayo, who with his persistent mother, Lesley, moved from Alabama to Budapest to receive treatment at the Petö Institute, received a great deal of attention a few years ago.[2]

Although the premise of the Petö program is not ostensibly gravity-based, I am convinced its success is because the children learn their movements in the upright position. This means they are using gravity, which is the primary stimulus for developing the sense of weight, distribution of weight during movement, and direction in propelling their weight forward. I have no doubt that improvement could be accelerated if the treatment included hypergravity—greater than 1G—on a centrifuge at the earliest possible age. Moving the legs back and forth in a walking motion could be mechanized so that even before a child would normally stand, he or she could experience motion at 1G or greater while lying down.

As a compromise, or in addition to other training, children with cerebral palsy or other motor handicaps can benefit from similar gravity stimulation with a "baby bounce" or "baby jump seat" type of exerciser (making sure that it includes an appropriate safety harness).[3] The joy such children show with this "toy seat" is testimony to its effectiveness.

The child's sensitivity or threshold to gravity may also be deficient depending on how long the child has been immobile. Increasing the intensity or frequency of the gravity stimulus during such physical therapy may initially be required. Using a centrifuge or some other device to do this may one day prove to be even more beneficial.

ADULT BRAIN INJURY

Stroke, aneurysm, tumor, disease, or trauma may damage brain centers or interrupt their lifeline to blood and oxygen supply. The brain is remarkably resilient and plastic. Given appropriate stimulation, involving gravity for motor coordination, it will bypass or reroute the nerve pathways to find ways of compensating for the damage suffered. The student daughter of a colleague at Stanford, whom we will call Emily, was run down by a car while trying to save her cat. The accident left her in a comatose state. Family and friends provided round-the-clock stimulation through talk, reading, and music. Weeks later, and against all odds, Emily regained consciousness. As soon as she could sit up, the next step in her healing were daily rides on Great America's roller coaster! Emily eventually regained some mobility and finished college.

VICTIMS OF SPINAL CORD INJURY ARE STARVED OF GRAVITY

Another common GDS case is those people who have been paralyzed by spinal cord injury, or by brain or neurological disorder. The spinal cord passes through the neck and back, is protected by bony vertebrae, and contains nerves that transport messages between the brain and the rest of the body. Individuals who are paralyzed, although surrounded by gravity—which, in fact, pins them to their wheelchair—cannot sense injury in their lower limbs below the point of trauma. Consequently, forced inactivity, together with an inability to sense and use gravity in their lower body, deprives them of the stimulus provided by loading their legs, hips, and lower spine with the body's weight. Just as we've seen happening with astronauts, leg muscles atrophy, joints stiffen, and bones become fragile. Equally, the inability to change position without help or to accelerate by running or walking affects stamina and the ability to regulate blood pressure. Feeling faint when sitting up was once thought to be the result of nerve damage. It is now clear that this is merely a consequence of being bed-bound. Studies have shown that upper body exercising corrects the tendency in these patients to faint on sitting up. Furthermore, acceleration, even while sitting in a wheelchair, stimulates the gravity sensors in their inner ear.

Individuals with these kinds of injuries who have the willpower to persevere may overcome many of these handicaps. They make the most of their upper body to stay remarkably fit. Building upper-body strength allows them to sit up and use their arms to transfer to the wheelchair. They may be seen whizzing around a basketball court, roaring down a ski slope, kayaking, or crossing the country at a pace that far outdoes many an able-bodied competitor. In recent decades, thousands of athletes with paralysis have raced in wheelchair marathons and competed in a

---

ACCESS ANYTHING: I CAN DO THAT!

Craig Kennedy's motto is "Go Anywhere, Do Anything." Paralyzed from the waist down at 23 when his spine was broken in a ski accident, Craig was faced with a choice—withdraw from life or make the most of what he had. After overcoming the physical trauma of his injury, he grappled with the emotional trauma of being unable to use his legs and the challenge of figuring out how he was going to take care of himself. Equipped with a positive attitude, he started thinking, "When am I going to try that new sport?" or "….this new adventure?" With his wife Andy, he formed the "Access Anything" company, whose mission is to improve accessibility for people with disabilities at lodging, transportation, recreation, and wilderness area facilities. Craig and Andy's passion is to encourage everyone to enjoy life through the sense of freedom that travel, adventure, and a "never give up" attitude make possible. Craig is still an avid skier, hitting the slopes in his specially designed equipment more than 80 days per season, and his latest sport challenge is kayaking.[5]

---

wide variety of sports in both summer and winter Paralympic Games. A remarkable example of one whose handicap does not hold him back from enjoying life is Itzhak Perlman. Considered one of the finest violinists of his generation, he overcame being struck down by polio at the age of four. Undaunted, he stuns the audience when negotiating the stage with braces and crutches. Perlman is also an enthusiastic proponent of wheelchair tennis.

MAINTAINING THE DISCONNECTED BODY

There may be much more that we have learned from space research that might help spinal cord injury (SCI) patients. Gravity acts on the body as a mechanical stimulus (see Chapter 3). The strain signals that arise in bone tissue during weight-bearing activities increase bone density of the lower limbs, while the absence of such signals is considered the main cause of the reduced bone mineral density in long bones that predisposes them to fractures. SCI patients belong to this class. They are plagued by hard-to-heal lower-limb bone fractures because they cannot feel where their lower limbs are positioned.

However unlikely, if Clinton Rubin's low-intensity, high-frequency vibration approach (a.k.a. Dynamic Motion; discussed in Chapter 3) indeed acts directly on lower-limb muscle and bone and does not require intact spinal neural access to the brain, then muscle integrity and bone density could theoretically be maintained with such vibration treatment. Studies are currently in progress at New York's Mount Sinai Medical Center that seek to answer this important question. This approach would provide much needed lower-body muscle and bone maintenance, not to mention enhanced repair of bone fractures.

Similar benefits from vibration therapy would be expected in patients whose spinal cord is not severed but whose motor cortex has suffered some injury from stroke. Vibration therapy might also help children and adults with cerebral palsy, or any other immobilizing condition. In fact, a study in children aged 4–19 years old with cerebral palsy or muscular dystrophy by Kathryn Ward and her colleagues at the University of Manchester found substantial improvement after treatment consisting of standing on the vibrating plate 10 minutes per day, five days a week for six months—about a 50 percent improvement in the bone density of their tibia.[6] The strain provided was 0.3G and the frequency was 90Hz. The strain, frequency and duration of exposure may vary depending on the condition of the patient.

Re-establishing Connections

Gravity therapy could possibly provide much more benefit than does mere maintenance were it to be applied soon after the SCI and before significant neural integrity beyond the point of injury in the lower body was lost. Some animal species, like salamanders, are capable of regenerating spinal cord connections after the cord is severed. The spinal cord-injured rat can recover some degree of mobility depending on the extent of the damage and the amount of weight-bearing activity generated after the injury.[7] Reggie Edgerton and his team at UCLA based their locomotor step-training approach in SCI humans on studies in SCI cats who regained the ability to step on a treadmill through full-weight locomotor training.[8] Recent experimental evidence provided by a group of researchers, led by Michael Sofroniew at UCLA, showed that SCI mice could essentially start walking again within eight to ten weeks, though not as well as before the injury, through the use of a process that diverted messages from the brain through shorter fibers and connections in the cord's center and around the damaged area to the limbs.[9]

To summarize, G-therapy—therapy with increasing gravity loads—involves getting gravity stimulation back into your life. It should benefit those who, for whatever reason, have developed a health problem from either being *less exposed to gravity's influence* or from *losing the ability to sense it.* This could be due to lifestyle, congenital, or developmental causes, or the result of injury or disease. It includes a very broad spectrum of neurological, metabolic, or even sports-related injuries resulting in forced inactivity, where gravity, hypergravity, or acceleration stimuli could promote healing. G-therapy is particularly important for speedy and proper rehabilitation.

Let's conclude this chapter with a look at some specific techniques researchers are developing for providing this G-therapy.

Hypergravity—Changing the Gravity Load

Centrifugation—Increasing the Load

A spinning centrifuge is the most reliable way of increasing the force of gravity on whoever rides it. Professors Larry Young and Tom Jarchow at MIT found that most people adapt in a short time to any discomfort caused by the intermittent repeated exposure to a short arm—2m radius—centrifuge spinning at 23 rpm (revolutions per minute). As you might expect from what you have read so far, such exposure should correct all those unpleasant consequences of living without gravity. However, research is continuing to determine exactly what the optimal G-prescription might be for individual problems.

We know from studies with animals that living for a few weeks on such a spinning centrifuge at 2G—twice Earth's gravity—has significant positive effects. The animals develop stronger muscles and bones. And, amazingly, they all become leaner. Mice, rats, rabbits, chickens, dogs, and monkeys all lose most of their body fat—especially the hard-to-lose abdominal fat. After eight weeks on a centrifuge at 2G, mice lost 55 percent of their body fat! This is not because they ate less or were more active. In fact, the opposite was true—the mice ate more and were less active! *Gravity, rather than activity or dieting, altered their metabolism to produce this leaner state.*

It is obviously not practical for humans to live continuously at 2G, or at any other level greater than Earth's 1G. However, even in these animal studies, it turns out that exposure to hypergravity was not continuous, after all. The centrifuge was stopped for one or two hours each day to clean it and replenish food and water. Because they are free to move within their cages, animals experience periods of activity and inactivity.

GET FIT WITHOUT MOVING A MUSCLE

A headline a few years from now might just read: "A new study shows that overweight people lose about as much muscle mass in 10 years—10 percent—as astronauts do on extended space missions. Now physicians are fighting fat with the NASA-inspired human centrifuge, a spinning platform that doubles the gravitational load on the body, stimulating metabolism and forcing muscles to contract. The person 'exercising' lies on a form-fitting pad, spins at 20 rpm for 10 minutes, and receives a benefit equivalent to an hour of weight lifting."

Would that not be great? But is it possible? There has as yet been no proof that you would become leaner when exposed to slightly higher levels of gravity on a centrifuge. But research has shown in animals that riding a centrifuge can kick-start metabolism, pump up the heart and circulation, increase bone density and muscle mass, and accelerate the healing of wounds and bone fractures. Imagine a time when you can lose fat and increase muscle while taking a fun spin on a centrifuge!

Does one need to live at 2G to derive this fat-mobilizing benefit, or will intermittent G exposure be as effective? We do not have the answer yet. Alternating high and low G exposures has proven to be the most effective mode of administering G in humans, but changes in stored fat have not been measured. Neither have there been any studies on humans with short bursts of slightly higher G to find out if they become leaner like the rabbits do. However, I am convinced that exposure to such bursts of hypergravity will prove effective in kick-starting metabolism. I predict that one day soon, centrifuges will be used to reduce body fat, particularly in obese individuals who may be unable to exercise.

And let's not forget all those otherwise healthy people who would like to get or stay strong and active in less time, without having to use 10 machines and 20 exercises. Being in hypergravity does the work for you since your muscles spontaneously contract, and your increased weight—without increasing your mass—stimulates bone strength.

Upright Loading

Increasing body weight by wearing removable loads around the ankles or wrists, or wearing a weighted vest during walking, has been used to strengthen muscles and, particularly, bones in those suffering from bone density loss. Weights have also been carried by those who wish to increase their stamina without increasing the duration of their activity or training.

Directional Brain Programming

Standing upright, even if the body weight is partially supported with a safety harness, has been extremely beneficial in children with various forms of brain injury—congenital, suffered at birth, or developed later. As mentioned earlier, the Pető Institute in Budapest, Hungary, uses this approach to train children with cerebral palsy and similar conditions to learn walking movements through repetitive motor activities, while standing upright. This means they are using gravity to learn how to sense and support their body weight during movement and as they propel their weight forward. As they move, their weight and its distribution provides feedback to their brain to set up appropriate networks.

This is an example where using *hypergravity* on a centrifuge should further accelerate the effectiveness of treatment by increasing the sensation of body weight at the feet while the child is lying down with its head towards the center of the centrifuge. As the child becomes accustomed to the rotation, its limbs could be moved back and forth in a walking motion by an attendant also riding the centrifuge, or moved automatically by a suitably designed walking or stepping machine.

Impact Loading

In children with brain injury, alternating loads greater than 1G can be provided by using a version of a "trampoline" suspended from an overhead spring, with the child seated in a harness, legs inserted through holes in the seat. By pushing off the ground, the child can bounce up and down. Children learn to enjoy the sensation of this device—which was developed as a toy—before they learn to walk, or even if they suffer disabilities. They derive fun and tremendous gravity value through directional, weight-loading impact and gravity sensor stimulation in their bare feet.

Cameron, diagnosed with *encephalomalacia,* the result of hypoxia at birth, is not an unusual case. His prognosis of cerebral palsy and developmental delays included feeding issues that required the use of a feeding tube for a while. He also had communication difficulties. He loved his "toy seat," jumping for hours in his playpen. As Cameron grew older, he used an adapted version that has been a huge help, not least because he loves it. More recently, he graduated to sitting on a special balance disc—discussed in Chapter 4 and below—that he enjoys, even as it stimulates gravity receptors in his buttocks and forces him to maintain better balance.

I see no reason why similar seated trampolines could not be useful for seniors who have trouble walking. Some personalized trampolines for home use are available commercially, but these are not seated, nor do they provide a safety harness. Though some have a partial safety rail for support, they are meant for those whose balance and strength is still fairly good. The ones who could really benefit from such a "bounce" device are those seniors in wheelchairs who need to strengthen leg muscles and bones and reinforce balance.

Inverted Loading or Antigravity

Relief from back pain may come from being suspended head downward on a board for 20–30 minutes. Sometimes referred to as antigravity, this technique uses gravity to shift the body's weight load from the feet to the head, as opposed to the normal upright head-to-toe direction. Needless to say, this must be done under proper supervision. It uses gravity to lengthen the spine and joints and relieve the pressure on the discs between the vertebrae. The person, lying on a board, is secured with straps, while the feet are placed into shoes attached to a crossbar or foot-plate as the board is tilted downwards. Alternately, a series of sessions is provided for $8,000, during which you are confined in a G-suit, primarily to minimize the risk of deep vein thrombosis and the tendency to faint on returning to the upright position, while you are tilted upside down and stretched. This stretching, not unlike old-fashioned traction techniques, lengthens the spine and provides temporary relief. However, once the patient is returned to the normal upright position and subject to their own weight, their symptoms recur, but there were those who have had this treatment claim "miraculous" relief and a few claim recovery.

When first introduced in the U.S.,[10] boots or ankle straps used for hanging upside-down were called Cuban or Gravity Boots, respectively, and there was no supporting board, which made them very unsafe, often resulting in back injuries. Current adaptations, such as the CX-900, are becoming popular among chiropractors for back pain treatment.

Vibration

As I described in Chapter 3, Clinton Rubin at State University of New York, in Stony Brook, has been playing with ways of "tricking" the body into thinking it is receiving a load-bearing strain in order to make bones stronger. He found that the kind of strain muscles continuously place on bones while a person is sitting or standing—strain that stimulates bone strength—is close to oscillations provided by vibration—very frequent but mild. He found that standing on a mildly vibrating platform for 10 to 20 minutes at the correct frequency stimulates bone mass and strength.

It has always been assumed that loading was essential to stimulating bone growth. However, recently, Rubin got even better results in mice without the need to load the bones by causing the mice to stand on them. He did this by applying, directly to the feet of the mice, extremely small oscillatory 0.6G accelerations at 45Hz for 20 minutes a day, five days a week. The results were spectacular—70 percent greater bone formation rates with both quality and quantity of newly formed bone improved as the result of the G-acceleration stimulus.

Needless to say, these findings must be confirmed in humans, but the results in mice are so dramatic that this approach of delivering the G stimulus shows excellent promise. Rubin explains these results as evidence of the existence of mechanosensors in bone-forming cells, whose job is to perceive and respond to acceleration G-signals. A recent review provides extensive discussion on the benefits of vibration.[11]

This mechanism may go beyond bone formation to a fundamental means by which gravity is transduced specifically to cells and tissues. The implications for those suffering from osteoporotic bone loss are huge, and the possibility that this is a generic mechanism for other systems is immense.

Stimulating Gravity Receptors

An alternative to increasing the gravity load is to work on increasing the sensitivity of gravity receptors by the use of techniques described in this section. Some forms of massage of the soles of the feet and buttocks could fall into this category, as well.

Balance Discs

A wide variety of inflated 12–15-inch balance discs with smooth, tactile surface bumps have appeared on the market for the development of balance skills and trunk strength. As described in Chapter 5, these resemble a flat, circular, air-filled cushion, except that the unevenness provided by the bumps forces the sitter to make continual small adjustments to maintain balance while sitting on the disc. Naturally, such continual adjustment allows the bumps to intermittently stimulate proprioceptors in the buttocks. Generally intended to be used for balance training or to provide a bit of exercise for healthy people who spend many hours sitting at a desk, they are turning out to have interesting potential in treatments.

During one of my talks to a group in Chapel Hill, an elementary school teacher in the audience shared that she had begun using such discs in her fifth-grade classroom with boys who were restless and could not concentrate. Boys sitting on these discs were more attentive and sat still longer than usual. No claims for Attention Deficit Disorder were made, but these discs appear to improve concentration in children.

The boy with cerebral palsy I mentioned earlier, Cameron, who is now seven, has his own balance disc. His mother says, "It brings nothing but smiles and talking when he gets on the disc. He always perks up, becomes more alert (eyes wide with awe and wonderment), and soon the kicking begins, along with the talking and it just becomes a party! He loves it." Cameron loves his swing in the backyard, as well. Some bells hung on the tree behind it jingle when he goes up high enough.

For a child like Cameron, every bit of gravity stimulation is therapy. Since he cannot move by himself, he cannot get enough stimulation in the course of the day to keep his gravity sensors tuned. I encouraged Cameron's mother to take him on a roller coaster, but the amusement park company would not allow it, so when they came to the next spinning ride, she did not ask. She just got on with him and he loved it! If Craig and Andy Kennedy's Access Anything organization (mentioned earlier in this chapter) has anything to do with it, the disabled will soon be enjoying these fantastic, health-promoting rides.

THE SWAY PLATFORM

A sway platform device called *dynamic posturography* was developed by NASA to test astronauts returning from space. It is a small computerized platform that tilts back and forth, on which the astronaut stands with eyes open or eyes closed. The degree of sway is used to evaluate the extent of balance and coordination deficit. In fact, it measures how well the body senses and is able to respond to the instability caused by standing on the platform. Because it is so sensitive, this sway test is now being used by the National Institute on Aging in its Baltimore Aging Longitudinal Study to detect the age at which the earliest onset of balance problems can be detected.

Wynford Dore, a British industrialist in Australia, picked up on this idea and put together a team to use the sway platform not as a test as originally designed, but in a treatment approach for his daughter, who suffered from severe chronic learning difficulties. His premise was that stimulation of the cerebellum—a part of the brain which coordinates movement and balance—by a series of balance and eye exercises would improve concentration and learning. "The unexpected breakthrough came when his company discovered that such programs initially used to treat dyslexia also had a powerful effect on ADHD," said Phil Mercer on BBC News, Sydney. The treatment is expensive, costing around $3,000, and takes up to 15 months to complete. Preliminary observations have been sufficiently interesting to merit further study, and these are apparently being conducted in the United Kingdom and Australia.[12]

HIPPOTHERAPY—RIDING THERAPY

Therapeutic riding for the sick and disabled makes use of horses to treat a variety of illnesses, along with accident and injury trauma of neurological origin. The horse's three-dimensional motion is the treatment tool for a wide array of cognitive, emotional, and behavioral disorders, such as autism, cerebral palsy, Parkinson's disease, multiple sclerosis, Down's syndrome, traumatic brain or spinal cord injury, stroke, ADHD, and learning or language disabilities. Even visual or hearing impairments, as well as emotional disorders such as depression, have been said to benefit.

Therapeutic riding is not new. It was first documented by the ancient Greeks when Orbassis of Lydia noted therapeutic effects of horseback riding in 600 b.c. A French physician in the 1870s began using horseback riding treatment for neurological disorders, concluding that the movements of the horse helped his patients' balance, posture, joints, and muscles. Danelle Kern, a physical therapist at Loma Linda University Medical Center and Childrens' Hospital in California, has her own seven-acre Therapeutic Riding Centre in Reche Canyon. She comments that "no machine has ever been invented to take the place of a horse's muscle groups, moving from side to side, forward and backward, and upward and downward. They closely mimic the human gait."

Critics dismiss it as alternative medicine with little scientific proof to back it. However, it is difficult to set up meaningful research designs because of the inexact nature of each treatment, complicated by variables such as different kinds of horses and instructors, as well as the broad range of conditions and ailments being treated.

Changing Posture

The simplest way to alternate the gravity load on the body is by changing posture. Most of us do this by getting up out of bed or from a chair or off the floor. Not only are bones and muscles stimulated, but this also does wonders for the development and regulation of blood pressure sensors. However, those who never developed these sensors, or lost them, or had their sensors lose sensitivity, experience problems with maintaining blood pressure. They can no longer respond reflexively to sitting up or standing with an appropriate rise in heart pumping, sufficient to protect them from the drop in blood pressure that could lead to fainting. Even if they do not faint and fall, they will feel unwell, weak, and possibly sweat or become nauseated.

Diabetics are prone to these symptoms, as are those with SCI, stroke, the elderly, and the generally less mobile. Ideally, practicing standing up often and deliberately is the simplest treatment. If one is unable to stand up unaided, an electrically operated chair that gently lifts a person up—a lift-chair—could help get the motion started. People who use these chairs may find they no longer need the chair after a while.

Changing posture "often" means every 15 to 20 minutes throughout the day. This interval allows the body time to ideally recover from the stimulus and response to each standing event before the next one. Aim for 30–35 posture changes a day. For those in nursing homes who are unable to stand on their own, an electric tilt-up bed—not a sit-up bed—could provide the desired daily G-dose of posture change. It is highly probable that patients following this regimen would regain the ability to stand up on their own and move about.

Now imagine a child with cerebral palsy or other brain injury at birth who has not had the benefit of alternating postural change that comes with normal development of movement and coordination. Such a child will not have developed the needed pressure reflex sensitivity to respond to sitting up or being held up. He or she may well feel faint, nauseous, unwell, weak, and may even vomit when sitting up, but how would one know? These children cannot communicate what they feel. Why would any parent or caregiver think these symptoms are not directly due to the brain injury and can be prevented? Why should this child be any more handicapped than necessary? Frequent changes in posture are the answer.

I am unaware of a commercial product that provides this type of treatment, but something simple could be rigged up. Watching able-bodied children playing on a seesaw, I wondered whether their less-able brother might not also enjoy and benefit from the ride, lying with suitably padded protection, his waist at the center of the seesaw! A steeper tilt up would be ideal, but it would be so much better if posture change were part of a game.

These are only a few examples of how understanding and using gravity and hypergravity is beginning to find its way into the treatment of musculoskeletal, bone, metabolic, cardiovascular, and neurological disorders. Infants and very young children have the most to gain, given the extraordinary plasticity of their nervous system.

Chapter 6 Notes

1. Edgerton, V. R., deLeon, R. L., Tillakaratne, N., Recktenwal, M. R., Hodgson, J. A., Roy, R. R. "Use-dependent plasticity in spinal stepping and standing." *Advances in Neurology: Neuronal Regeneration, Reorganization and Repair*, F. J. Seil (ed.) 72: 233–248, Philadelphia: Lippincott-Raven Publishers, 1997.

2. Source: "Mind and Muscle: Petö Institute brings hope to kids with cerebral palsy." Aug. 18, 2004. http://www.cbsnews.com/stories/2004/02/24/60II/main601944.shtml (accessed 10/29/07).

3. http://www.rightstart.com/search/result/?q=exersaucer; see also "Johnny Jump-Up" http://www.nextag.com/evenflo-johnny-jump-up/search-html.

4. "What's New in Neurogenesis," An Interview with Fred H. Gage, Ph.D. The Dana Foundation, 2007. http://www.thedanafoundation.org

5. Source: Craig and Andrea Kennedy, "Access Anything," http://www.ckconsultingonline.com/about.html(accessed 1/24/08).

6. Ward, K., Alsop, C., Caulton, J., Rubin, C., Adams, J., Mughal, Z. "Low magnitude mechanical loading is osteogenic in children with disabling conditions." *J Bone Min Res* 19:360–367, 2004.

7. Engesser, C. C., Ichiyama, R., Nefas, A. L., Hill, M. A., Edgerton, V. R., Cotna, C. W., Anderson, A. J. {"Wheel running following spinal cord injury improves locomotor recovery and stimulates serotonergic fiber growth." *Eur J Neurosci* 25:1931–1939, 2007.

8. Edgerton, R. V., Roy, R. R., Hodgson, J. A., Day, K., Weiss, J., Harkema, S. J., Dobkin, B., Garfinkel, A., Konigsberg, E., Kozlovskaya, I. "How the Science an Engineering of Spaceflight Contribute to Understanding the Plasticity of Spinal Cord Injury." *Acta Astronautica* 47 (1):51–62, 2000.

9. Courtine, G., Song, B., Roy, R. R., Zhong, H., Herman, J. E., Ao, Y., Qi, J., Edgerton, V. R., Sofroniew, M. V. "Recovery of supraspinal control of stepping via indirect propriospinal relay connections after spinal cord Injury." *Nature Med.*, Pub Med. 6 January, 2008.

10. Source:http://www.comfortchannel.com/level.itml/icOid/765; See also *UC Berkeley Wellness* Letter from Sept 2001: http://www.wellnessletter.com/html/wl/2001/wlAskExperts0901.html.

11. Totosy de Zepetnek, J. O., Giangregorio, B., Craven, C. "Whole-body vibration as potential intervention for people with low bonemineral density and osteoporosis: A review." *J Rehab Res Dev* 46(4):529–542, 2009.

12. Source: Phil Mercer, http://www.BBCNews.com 2007; see also http://www.dore.co.uk/LearningDifficulties/Default.aspx (accessed 1/24/08).

Epilogue

The state of health in the world is deteriorating. In the United States, two out of every three people are unhealthy. This alarming trend must be stemmed and reversed, or it will cripple personal health, national vitality, and resources. Something needs to be done.

The culprit is neither a virus nor a toxic pollutant. The enemy is a transformation in lifestyle that probably saw its beginnings with urbanization during the Industrial Revolution. A change from physically working the land and needing hearty meals was now followed by standing in factory assembly lines while eating just as much, particularly carbohydrates. This shift accelerated in the 20th century, when even more sedentary forms of work were accompanied by eating more food than required by the body. And food itself changed with the widescale use of canning and preservation, followed by the introduction of freezers and the addition of chemicals to maintain food crispness and enhance its color appeal. Affluence and cars for most families diminished physical activity even more.

The electronic revolution followed. Gadgets, automation, instant communications on a global scale, and home entertainment eliminated what few healthful activities remained. Yet appetite has not decreased since the time of the hearty farmer's breakfast. From the school yard to the comfort of your home, advertising, packaging, and instant food delivered to your door provide relentless stimulation, offering countless food choices rich in salt, sugar, and fat that further trigger brain appetite centers.

Though the quality of medical care is better than ever, its cost is becoming prohibitive. The solution is to motivate the return of healthy lifestyle practices. But the medical system often stands in the way. Doctors are trained to treat patients, not to prevent them from ever getting sick. The

Hippocratic approach, interpreted liberally, of allowing nature to heal itself with minimum interference is no longer common practice in our pill-happy culture. But no course in preventive health care is offered in medical school, and a master's degree in public health is the closest we come to preventive health care education.

Healthy people are neglected by our medical system and often penalized for not using doctors' services. They pay the same premiums, but, unlike the sick, get no tax break on medical expenses if they do not exceed a minimum threshold. There are no financial incentives to remain healthy. So how can the unhealthy be motivated to return to good health?

If the poor health epidemic of today is due to lifestyle, then our present dire situation should be reversible by a change in that lifestyle. We achieved something similar with anti-smoking campaigns. The Space Age gave us many of the modern technologies that encourage a sedentary lifestyle resulting in obesity and poor health, but it also revealed the problem's cause as well as its solution. We cannot return to our old ways, abolish technology, and give up modern conveniences. But we can choose to use gravity or let it drag us down. This is the secret that living in the weightlessness of space revealed.

This book is a manual for preventive health care and a guide to living a natural, health-sustaining lifestyle. When correctly used, the gravity vector is a great healer. Moreover, it's a great source of fun! Look at a child playing and you will note that every fun game, every position, challenges the gravity vector. This vigorous enjoyment of gravity should not end in childhood—it is needed throughout life to promote and reinforce the complex circuitry and systems of the body. So be a child again. Play.

Space research points out that the body senses and responds to the gravity stimulus best when the signals are frequent, low intensity, stop-start movements experienced throughout the day. This book challenges the conventional wisdom that structured, intense, once-a-day exercise is all you need to replace being active the rest of the time. Its message is simple: If you want to remain healthy and strong for life on Earth, keep doing things, a variety of things, all day, 365 days a year.

It's up to you. Success is a question of attitude, and attitude that should be based on the desire to remain healthy. Your body is your personal responsibility—not your country's, nor your insurance company's, nor even your doctor's. Take action. Why wait to get sick before you decide to be healthy?

Appendix
Health Assets Questionnaire

Congratulations on taking this time to invest in yourself. Just as people have 401(k)s and other investments which reflect their financial well-being, this brief questionnaire will help you assess your current health assets. Whatever your age and state of physical and mental health, by making health-conscious investments in yourself today, you will build up reserves that you can rely on in the future.

Read the following statements and answer as truthfully as possible by circling the appropriate number:

1. How well do you feel in terms of your health at this moment?

1	2	3	4	5
Extremely unwell—serious health concerns and pain which impact my independence and outlook	Unwell—suffering complications and pain from medical conditions	Okay—few aches and pains or moderate health concerns which I manage most of the time	Generally well—no serious concerns, active and independent	Great—no complaints!

2. When do you have the most energy?

1	2	3	4	5
Evening	Late afternoon	Midday	Mid-morning	Early morning

3. How satisfied are you with your looks?

1	2	3	4	5
Dissatisfied	Somewhat dissatisfied	Happy with some features, unhappy with others	Mostly satisfied	Very happy

4. How would you rate your eating habits?

1	2	3	4	5
I skip meals, eat fast and fatty foods, often on the go	I eat at irregular times, not the healthiest choices	I make some healthy as well as some unhealthy choices	I eat mostly healthier meals at the dining table	I eat regularly scheduled, consistently healthy meals

5. How much water do you drink per day? (one cup = 8 ounces)

1	2	3	4	5
1 cup	2–3 cups	4–5 cups	6–7 cups	8 or more cups

6. How well do you manage your weight?

1	2	3	4	5
I'm usually more than 25 pounds over my ideal body weight	I am 20–25 pounds over my ideal body weigh	I am within 10–20 pounds of my ideal body weight	I am within 10 pounds of my ideal body weight	I maintain my ideal body weight

7. How well do you manage your stress?

1	2	3	4	5
I feel anxious and overwhelmed most of the time and don't know how to find relief	I find myself trying to cope mostly by eating, drinking, or taking my aggression out on others	Sometimes I feel overwhelmed, and at other times I am better able to cope	I manage the stresses in my life fairly well most of the time	I feel little stress in my life

8. How well do you manage your time?

1	2	3	4	5
I am rarely on schedule and never seem to get things done on time	I am sometimes on schedule. I have trouble prioritizing commitments and I always seem to have more to do	I move between good and bad days, sometimes able to accomplish goals but other times not	Most of the time I organize my day well and accomplish the day's goals	I am regularly able to organize my time to accomplish each day's goals

9. How would you describe your sleep?

1	2	3	4	5
I have trouble falling asleep, wake up frequently, and nod off during the day	I rarely sleep soundly and feel tired most days.	I may fall asleep easily but wake up and have trouble going back to sleep. I sometimes sleep through the night and wake up feeling rested.	I often fall asleep easily, wake up occasionally, but generally feel rested	I fall asleep easily, sleep soundly, and wake up refreshed

10. How would you describe your level of activity?

1	2	3	4	5
I spend most of the day sitting or lying down	I sit for hours at a stretch and am not very active	I am somewhat active, exercise occasionally, and sit most of the rest of the day	I exercise 2–3 times a week, get up often, and make a point of being active	In addition to exercising regularly, I am active throughout the day

11. How would you describe your support network?

1	2	3	4	5
I have little contact with others and no one I can call on when in need	I have a few friends whom I rarely see; I am alone much of the time	I have some friends whom I value, and we communicate and see each other from time to time	I have a few friends and family members on whom I can rely, and with whom I often talk or socialize	I have many good friends, neighbors, and extended family on whom I can rely and with whom I frequently talk or socialize

12. How would you describe your balance?

1	2	3	4	5
I have difficulty standing or walking unsupported	I lose my balance quickly and have to sit even for basic things like putting my socks on	I often need to lean against something to get dressed	I can easily put my slacks and socks on standing up	I can comfortably stand on either leg for one minute or more

13. In an average weekday how much time are you devoting to yourself?

1	2	3	4	5
Almost none at all	I am so busy with commitments, I'm lucky to get more than 30 minutes for my own enjoyment	Most days I am able to spend adequate time but I wish I had a little more	More than 3 hours—I have plenty of time for my desired activities	Most of the day—I have few other commitments

14. What is your age?

1	2	3	4	5
91 or older	70–89 years	45–69 years	26–44 years	25 or younger

15. Which profile best describes your alcoholic drinking habits?

1	2	3	4	5
I drink every day; I need it to function	Almost every day I have three or more drinks	More days than not I have a drink or two Or I am an alcoholic and don't drink now	Some days I enjoy one and sometimes two drinks	I drink the occasional glass of beer or wine Or I don't drink at all

16. How many cigarettes do you smoke per day?

1	2	3	4	5
A pack or more	Daily, less than a pack	Most days, less than 10 Or I used to smoke regularly but quit	I smoke a cigarette once in a while	never

Subtotal (tally your points for the above questions): _____

Add 4 points if you are male and 5 if you are female _____

Total number of points _____

What is your health credit rating?

If you scored…

72–80: Your health portfolio is diversified and well-funded! You are making wise decisions today which are an investment in your lifelong vitality and independence.

59–71: You are making sound health investments. Small improvements in the way you manage your health today can result in a longer, more energetic and independent future. Keep it up.

46–58: Your health investments could use some attention. There are small but important steps you can take to make a difference right away, as well as better invest in your future.

33–45: Your state of health is compromised. You would significantly benefit from learning how to make adjustments to your daily habits.

32 or less: Your state of health is poor. If you are 55 or younger, the choices you are making are compromising your health today as well as your future ability to remain independent. This is the time to act! If you're not doing so already, consult with a physician or other health professional(s) in order to identify your risk areas and ways to address them.

Index

insulin levels 37
insulin resistance 80
intensity 56
International Space Station 14, 18, 80
Internet 41
inversion 70
Ireland 35
irritability 20
isolation 24
isometric 75, 78
isometric exercise 25, 82, 92
isotonic 75

J

JAMA 68
Jarchow, Tom 104
jet-lag 17
jitterbug 67
joba 89, 90
joints 58, 59, 63, 90, 99, 102, 107, 111
jumping 54, 70, 86
jumping jacks 71

K

Kansas 91
kayaking 70
Kegels 25, 82
Kennedy, Andy 102, 110
Kennedy, Craig 102, 110
Kennedy Space Center 91
Kern, Danelle 111
KickStart 26
kidney failure 24
kidney stones 15, 17
Knapp, Charles 92
Korfmacher, George 34, 87

L

Landy 76
Langer, Ellen 44
leg muscles 67, 72, 89, 102
legs 69
leucine 86
Levine, James 36
lift-chair 112
lifting 44
ligaments 58, 59
lipase 37
lipotoxicity 37
load-bearing strain 108
locomotion 16
locomotor step-training 104
Loma Linda University Medical Center and Childrens' Hospital 111
Lou Gehrig's disease 5, 21
low density lipoproteins (LDL) 37
lower-body muscle 103
lower limbs 103
low-gravity existence 4
low-intensity activity 41, 53, 55
lung circulation 99

M

Maazel, Loren 68
"mall-walkers" group 72
Manhattan, Kansas 91
marathon runners 85
marathons 75
Mars 11, 93

Masai Barefoot Technology (MBT) 90, 91
mass 11
Matsushita Electric Industrial Co. 90
Mayo, Blaine 100
Mayo Clinic 36
Mayo, Lesley 100
mechanical signals 40, 41
mechanosensors 108
Medical Veritas 98
Mehta, Zubin 68
menopause 20
Mercer, Phil 110
Mercury spacecraft 8, 13, 14
metabolic diseases 36
metabolic disorders 112
metabolic energy 76
metabolism 14, 72, 75, 80, 85, 86, 90, 93, 98, 105, 106
metabolites 37
Minnesota 36
MIT 104
mitochondria 35, 36
mobile-active 10
mobility, limited 21
mobilizer muscles 55
mobilizer muscle system 93
mobilizers 34, 52
moon 11, 13
moon face 15
Morley, George 98
Morrell, Stephen 9
motion sickness 56
motorbike 91
motor coordination 101
motor cortex 103

About the Author

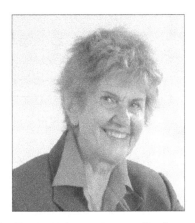

JOAN VERNIKOS, PH.D., is a pioneering medical research scientist who has conducted seminal studies in space medicine, inactivity physiology, stress, and healthy aging. Born in Alexandria, Egypt, in 1934, Vernikos received her Ph.D. in pharmacology at the University of London and became a researcher at the NASA Ames Research Center in 1964. She was a foundational figure of space medicine research and served as Life Sciences Director at the NASA Ames Research Center from 1986 to 1993 and Director of the Life Sciences Division at NASA headquarters from 1993 to 2000.

In her research at NASA, Vernikos spearheaded groundbreaking medical studies on the effects of weightlessness on health. Vernikos' NASA research on the health effects of weightlessness helped establish the scientific causal relationship between sedentary living, rapid aging and poor health.

Vernikos has been twice winner of NASA's Exceptional Leadership Award, and has also received NASA's Exceptional Scientific Achievement Award, the Melbourne Boynton Award from the American Astronautical Association, the Strughold Award in Space Medicine from the American Aerospace Medical Association, the Jeffries Award from the American Institute of Aeronautics and Astronautics, the Lifetime Achievement Award from Women in Aerospace, and numerous other academic and scientific awards.

Knowledge for healthy living from Quill Driver Books

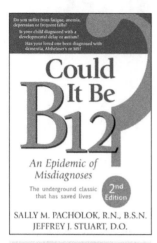

$14.95 ($16.95 Canada)

Could It Be B12?

An Epidemic of Misdiagnoses Second Edition
by Sally M. Pacholok, R.N., B.S.N., and
Jeffrey J. Stuart, D.O.

The underground classic that sparked a patients' rebellion and saved lives! *Could It Be B12?* reveals the facts about a health crisis most doctors don't know exists—the chronic misdiagnosis of vitamin B12 deficiency. If you or your loved ones have been diagnosed with Alzheimer's disease, dementia, multiple sclerosis, depression, fatigue, mental illness, frequent falls, forgetfulness, or other disorders, B12 deficiency may be the underlying cause. *Could It Be B12?* gives you the knowledge to take control of your health.

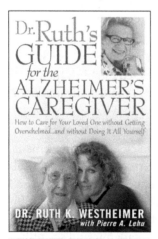

$16.95 ($18.95 Canada)

Dr. Ruth's Guide for the Alzheimer's Caregiver

How to Care for Your Loved One without Getting Overwhelmed ... and without Doing It All Yourself
by Dr. Ruth K. Westheimer
with Pierre A. Lehu

America's most-trusted sex therapist brings much-needed help to overburdened caregivers! *Dr. Ruth's Guide for the Alzheimer's Caregiver* presents coping strategies for both the practical problems and emotional stresses of Alzheimer's care. Dr. Ruth shows you how to avoid caregiver burnout; get effective support from family and friends; deal effectively with doctors, care providers and facilities.

Available from bookstores, online bookstores, and QuillDriverBooks.com, or by calling toll-free 1-800-345-4447.